The Essential Guide to Public Health and Health Promotion

Designed to help readers develop the practical skills needed to become effective public health practitioners, this concise text gives a highly accessible overview of the theory and practice of public health and health promotion.

The book covers a comprehensive range of key topics, beginning with a discussion of theoretical models and approaches to public health, before addressing important issues such as equality, health education and governmental policy. It also offers readers:

- Information on health needs assessment, including how to research, plan and evaluate practice with individual clients or population groups.
- Methods of helping people with motivation for behaviour change, building rapport, ongoing support, and signposting to services.
- The role of communities in improving health and how to support local populations.

In light of the Covid-19 pandemic, this 2nd edition has been updated with new material around vaccination and communicable disease and includes expanded coverage of mental health issues. There's also a new 'reflective thinking' feature to encourage a more critical approach.

The Essential Guide to Public Health and Health Promotion, 2nd edition is the ideal starting point for all those new to working or studying in the area, whatever their professional or academic background.

Susan R. Thompson has worked in the field of public health and health promotion for over 30 years within nursing, health promotion services and academia. She holds a master's degree in Public Health and has been an academic since 2005. In addition to this publication, she has published a range of articles and delivered international conference presentations and workshops. She is a trustee and board member of the Institute of Health Promotion and Education, an international body which seeks to support health promoters in their work and contribute to and lobby for policy change in the field of health promotion and public health.

The Essential Guide to Public Health and Health Promotion

Second Edition

Susan R. Thompson

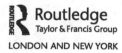
Routledge
Taylor & Francis Group

LONDON AND NEW YORK

Cover image: Getty Images VISION4RY-L4NGU4GE

First published 2023
by Routledge
4 Park Square, Milton Park, Abingdon, Oxon OX14 4RN

and by Routledge
605 Third Avenue, New York, NY 10158

Routledge is an imprint of the Taylor & Francis Group, an informa business

British Library Cataloguing-in-Publication Data
A catalogue record for this book is available from the British Library

Library of Congress Cataloging-in-Publication Data
Names: Thompson, Susan R. (Susan Rosemary), 1961- author.
Title: The essential guide to public health and health promotion / Susan R. Thompson.
Description: 2nd edition. | Abingdon, Oxon ; New York, NY : Routledge, 2023. |
Includes bibliographical references and index.
Identifiers: LCCN 2023002063 | ISBN 9780415813075 (hardback) | ISBN
9780415813082 (paperback) | ISBN 9780203068328 (ebook)
Subjects: LCSH: Public health. | Health promotion.
Classification: LCC RA425 .T46 2023 | DDC 362.1--dc23/eng/20230420
LC record available at https://lccn.loc.gov/2023002063

ISBN: 978-1-032-53293-6 (hbk)
ISBN: 978-1-032-13602-8 (pbk)
ISBN: 978-1-003-41132-1 (ebk)

DOI: 10.4324/9781003411321

Typeset in Sabon
by KnowledgeWorks Global Ltd.

Contents

Figures and Tables

Figures

Tables

Contributor Biographies

Jane Bethea is a consultant in Public Health for Nottinghamshire Healthcare NHS Foundation Trust and Training Programme Director for East Midlands Public Health training. Her professional interests are around vulnerable adults and improving outcomes for those experiencing a range of complex needs. She is the lead for Severe Multiple Disadvantage in Nottingham City and is closely involved in the City's Changing Futures programme. Other interests include reducing alcohol-related harm and improving outcomes for people experiencing co-existing substance use and mental health issues. She is passionate about her home city of Nottingham, with particular interests in the City's long and fascinating history.

David Charnock is an associate professor in Learning Disability Nursing at the University of Nottingham. His interests include health promotion and public health, partnership working and co-production with vulnerable groups, gender and identity. Before joining the University, David was employed in a number of senior roles for a large mental health and learning disabilities NHS trust, managing both community nursing and allied health services. Following the completion of his PhD studies in 2013, he has continued to develop his research interests using innovative methods to facilitate the involvement of people with a learning disability in projects about their lives.

Katriona Cheng is a registered adult nurse and Specialist Community Public Health Nurse and spent many years working with children and their families before beginning her career in academia. As a Health Visitor, she visited families to promote their health, well-being, growth and development, supporting children to have the best start in life and helping families access relevant and timely support. She developed significant safeguarding and multidisciplinary experience which led to an interest in the long-term impacts of adverse childhood experiences. She holds a master's degree in Public Health and now teaches across nursing, midwifery and the master's degree in Public Health programmes of the University of Nottingham. She is a fellow of the Higher Education Academy and is Deputy Safeguarding Lead for the School.

Matthew Horrocks is an assistant professor of Mental Health and Psychological Therapies at the University of Nottingham. Matt is a qualified Cognitive Behavioural Psychotherapist and Person-Centred Counsellor. Matt has worked in NHS primary care and mental health services for 20 years and continues to maintain clinical practice whilst contributing to the training and supervision of CBT therapists and mental health nurses at the University of Nottingham.

Mo Lockwood is a registered nurse and member of the Motivational Interviewing Network of Trainers. She has over 30 years' experience of working with people of all ages and backgrounds, across a broad spectrum of health-related settings. The majority of her career has been spent in the field of Public Health and Specialist Health Promotion, working to reduce health inequalities and improve health outcomes on a population and individual basis. Following her completion of an internationally recognised training in 2003 by Drs. William Miller and Stephen Rollnick, she has delivered MI training to a diversity of practitioners in the fields of education, health and well-being and social care. Mo also works as a specialist sexual health practitioner..

Vanessa McFarlane has worked in Health Promotion in the UK for over 25 years, with expertise in ethnic minority, sexual and young people's health. She is the chief executive of Mariposa Education & Training, an agency delivering relationship and sex education training to youth organisations. She is also a life coach working with adults and young people.

Patricia Owen is the President of the Institute of Health Promotion and Education and has had a long career in nursing, educating and promoting health. As President and a Trustee on the Board of the Institute of Health Promotion and Education, she works to promote health in its broadest sense with colleagues and members from around the UK and internationally. Her work with Health Education England on leadership learning in the pre-registration health curricula resulted in the development of national guidelines identifying strategies to build resilience in learner nurses and developing leadership learning. Patricia was Head of the School of Nursing and Midwifery at Keele University and since retirement from this role is Emeritus Professor of Nursing at Keele University and Director of Academic Health Consultancy Ltd.

Susan R. Thompson (Main Author) has worked in the field of public health and health promotion for over 30 years within nursing, health promotion services and academia. She holds a master's degree in Public Health and has been an academic since 2005. In addition to this publication, she has published a range of articles and delivered international conference presentations and workshops. She is a trustee and board member of the Institute of Health Promotion and Education, an international body which seeks to support health promoters in their work and contribute to and lobby for policy change in the field of health promotion and public health.

Michelle Turner is a diabetes specialist nurse, general practice nurse and physical activity clinical champion for the Office of Health Improvement and Disparity on the UK Moving Health Care Professionals Programme. She is a non-medical prescriber. She is a member of the Institute of Health Promotion and Education and the British Society of Lifestyle Medicine and is currently studying for a diploma with the American College of Lifestyle Medicine. She has experience in school nursing and palliative care and is now working on a pilot project of group consultations for people with diabetes in her Primary Care Network.

Oliver Wilkinson-Dale is a manager in the Public Health Team at Nottingham City Council. He qualified as a social worker in 2017 and worked as a social worker with people experiencing homelessness in Nottingham before moving to work in Public Health. He currently works promoting access to vaccinations for vulnerable groups and also coordinates the drug-related death review process for Nottinghamshire. He retains a professional interest supporting people experiencing complex needs and homelessness.

Foreword by Professor Patricia Owen

Some of the challenges to health that populations must contend with have changed fundamentally in recent years and, certainly, following the recent global Coronavirus pandemic. However, other problems facing populations, including the impact of inequality and poverty on health, remain stubbornly consistent over decades. These complex and sometimes seemingly insurmountable issues affecting health continue to require a coherent, evidence-based and creative approach to work towards resolutions. Therefore, a second edition of The Essential Guide to Health Promotion and Public Health is not only most welcome to practitioners and those learning the craft, but also a necessity. The skills, approaches and practicalities of promoting health, preventing ill health and assuring good public health in these uncertain times surely demonstrate that practitioners are an important key to good health for all.

This book covers all those fundamental areas which support high standards of health promoting practice. One of these key areas is understanding the concept of health itself from different perspectives and cultures and Chapter 1 identifies some of the frames of reference which practitioners need to consider when working with local, regional and national populations. How can one support individuals and groups to better health without first understanding what their view of health is?

We know which diseases are the main killers in our society today and Chapters 2 and 3 offer a comprehensive summary of these in order for practitioners to consider the contexts and broader views that inform prevention and health promotion in these areas. Obviously, in the UK, the National Health Service (NHS) still undertakes a mainly medical approach to disease prevention, but here in these chapters, other perspectives are considered and understanding of the complex societal dilemmas that affect health is laid bare.

Another fundamental area that is addressed early in the book is the challenge of how practitioners can promote health. Using information from Chapters 4–7, the practitioner will be able to assess the problems being faced, decide which approach to take to tackle the issue, consider which models help explain it and then in Chapter 8 start to plan a programme of health promoting activity. There are excellent case studies exemplified in this chapter which will support practice development in areas such as debates around promoting the health of the homeless.

Using appropriate evidence, primary data and secondary epidemiological data drives the best health promoting approaches to undertake and throughout the book, the importance of using current and high-ranking evidence is evident. When working with any group or community understanding the related statistics, local data, epidemiological studies and literature are fundamental to focussing on solutions. Building on the context of the discussion in Chapter 1, it is important to consider particular issues affecting different and diverse communities. Culture and ethnicity are significant aspects of health promoting and public health practice and practitioners need to understand these from the viewpoint of the communities themselves. Chapter 9 supports this work.

The Coronavirus pandemic highlighted the importance of our mental well-being, as people across the world endured isolation, grief and enforced estrangement from loved ones. Children and young people were affected by school closure and their reliance on technology was not always best placed to promote healthy relationships. Work to build mental health capacity, therefore, is a priority globally and methods to promote mental health are discussed in Chapter 10 with a particular focus on the ways cognitive behavioural therapy can support young people.

We know the marginalised and vulnerable often have poorer health outcomes and struggle more than others with achieving positive health, both individually and in society. The neighbourhood that supports these people often throws up many challenges to positive health, and it is important that those with learning disabilities are considered in Chapter 11. Those people with learning disabilities not only often struggle to navigate the complex health and social care system that should be in place to support them, but also have particular needs in relation to how their health can be sustained and improved. This chapter is immensely important in helping practitioners make their own practice effective for this group of people.

We know the importance of early years in setting the building blocks for a healthy life. Whether this is physical, emotional, or mental health. A focus on promoting health for children and young people is a priority for a healthy future society. Chapter 12 discusses aspects of health promotion for children and young people. As children spend many of their 'awake' hours at school, as a prospective health promoting setting, consideration of how schools can foster the health of children is salient.

Government guidelines around the world vary as to the amount of physical activity one should undertake to support health and prevent disease, but the World Health Organization (WHO) suggests that adults between the ages of 18 and 64 years should undertake at least 150–300 minutes of moderate-intensity aerobic activity throughout a week (WHO 2020). Chapter 13 helps the health promoting practitioner to consider why this is important and discusses approaches to enable individuals, communities and groups to achieve this target and to reduce sedentary lifestyles.

I began this foreword by confirming that there have been unprecedented recent challenges to health as well as continued seemingly intractable health issues affecting us all. In the concluding chapter, these are considered in further detail, especially some of those larger challenges, e.g. coronavirus, AMR, air pollution and climate change. Although these difficulties may appear unresolvable, by working with the methods and approaches outlined in this book and with will and resource, we could go a long way towards improving health for individuals and communities in years to come.

Professor Patricia Owen
President – The Institute of Health Promotion and Education
Emeritus Professor of Nursing, Keele University, Staffordshire, UK

Reference

World Health Organization. (2020). *WHO guidelines on physical activity and sedentary behaviour* [Online]. Geneva: WHO. Available at https://apps.who.int/iris/bitstream/handle/10665/336656/9789240015128-eng.pdf?sequence=1&isAllowed=y [accessed 16 November 2022].

1   What Is Health?

Susan R. Thompson

Health is a term used widely in societies. Asking about someone's health is one of the commonest forms of greeting worldwide. Yet, we take little time to consider exactly what is meant by the term health. It is argued that health is in fact a social construct and its meaning differs from society to society and from individual to individual, depending on cultural values and norms, personal experiences and attitudes (Barry and Yull 2021; Conrad and Barker 2010; O'Reilly and Lester 2016).

Definitions of Health

The World Health Organization (WHO) has defined health as '*a complete state of physical, mental and social well-being, and not merely the absence of disease or infirmity*' (WHO 1986). This seems like a distant possibility, as it is doubtful if any individual can say that they remain in such a blessed state for any significant period of time, if at all. However, this definition was revolutionary when it was first proposed as it acknowledged that health should not be seen as purely a biological status but one which encompasses psychological and social health as well. A more nuanced definition is Bircher's (2005, p. 1) who defines health as '*a dynamic state of well-being characterized by a physical and mental potential, which satisfies the demands of life commensurate with age, culture, and personal responsibility*'. This takes into account how levels of good health will naturally vary with age and individual expectations. The way we view health varies depending on our individual expectations, circumstances, experiences, age, gender and other factors such as societal influences, ethnicity and culture (Green et al. 2019; Warwick-Booth and Cross 2018).

Critical Thinking

Take a moment to think about how you view health.
Do you consider it at all? Or maybe only when you are ill?
Do you expect good health?
Do you think of health mainly in physical terms?
Have your perceptions of health changed as you grew older?

DOI: 10.4324/9781003411321-1

Models of Health

The Biomedical Model

Within western societies, the biomedical model of health prevails as the dominant model of health and until recently was largely unquestioned. Within this model, a disease is seen as a defined state experienced by the body as a result of a pathological condition which is either temporary (curable) or permanent (incurable). In the biomedical model of health, the mind and the body are seen as separate; the body is viewed as a functioning machine with all disease being explained by the physical working of the body which, if a disease is present, will need repairing (Farre and Rapley 2017). The biomedical model of health is also a very intervention-ist model which is forever developing new techniques, tests and treatments to achieve a cure or alleviate symptoms (Nettleton 1995). Biomedicine works from a pathogenic (origins of disease) focus, emphasising risk factors and defining normality and abnormality. Treatment of individuals is carried out by health professionals, primarily doctors who perform tests, diagnose disease and prescribe treatment, either medication or surgery. Qualitative evidence (given by lay people or produced through academic research) generally has a lower status as knowledge than quantitative evidence (Wade and Halligan 2004). It is incontrovertible that the biomedical model has had its successes, and diagnosis and treatment of disease based on this model is largely effective, as the worldwide eradication of smallpox has shown. However, it is not infallible and over the years the model has been evolving away from its strict origins. The biomedical model of health has traditionally played up its curative success and down-played the negative consequences or side effects of some of its treatments. Medical interven-tions can do harm as well as good. Overuse of antibiotic therapy, for example, has caused bacterial resistance, as in the case of the growth of Methicillin-resistant *Staphylococcus aureus* (MRSA). There has been a growing awareness even in the medical profession that there are problems with over-medicalisation (Wade and Halligan 2004). Over-diagnosis and unneces-sary treatment do occur which can lead to wasted resources, heightened patient anxiety and iatrogenesis which is harm caused by medical interventions (Bmj.com 2015).

Biopsychosocial Model of Health

First described by the psychiatrist George Engel in 1977 (Engel 1977), this model sought to in-corporate social, psychological and emotional factors in diagnosis and treatment. It recognises that illness cannot be studied or treated in isolation from the social and cultural environment. The model expects doctors and other health care workers to acknowledge people's circum-stances. Heart disease and obesity, for example, are linked epidemiologically to ethnicity and poverty and, therefore, cannot be explained simply in terms of individual self-responsibility and willpower. Rather, definitions of health within a biopsychosocial model consider the way in which people negotiate their way through environmental, social and informational influ-ences. These also consider issues such as improving access to health services and reducing health inequalities as a legitimate and appropriate function of health service provision and respect qualitative research. It is the biopsychosocial model which now forms the basis of western health care (Henningsen 2015; Ventres and Frankel 2021; Weston 2005).

Salutogenic Model

Salutogenesis is the concept of positive health. This model, developed by sociologist Aaron Antonovsky, focuses on how and why people stay well. Therefore, it is quite a move away from the biomedical model which focuses on illness. The Salutogenic model looks at the relationship between stressors (such as lack of social support, poverty, unstable environment, sense of self-worth, etc.) and health (Antonovsky 1979, 1996; Mittelmark and Bauer 2022). It concentrates on the way that we feel and our circumstances and how these can influence our stress levels, which may lead to ill health, both physical and psychological. It proposed the concept of ideal balance, people not being under loaded or overloaded, neither bored nor overly stressed (Mittelmark and Bauer 2022; Polhius et al. 2020).

Other Models of Health

Cultures around the world define health differently. Australian Aboriginal people generally define health as not just the well-being of the individual but also the social, emotional, spiritual and cultural well-being of the whole community (NHMRC 1996). This is very different from the individualised western way of viewing health. Believers in traditional Chinese medicine think that the body holds a vital force of energy the Qi (pronounced 'chee'). For the body to remain healthy, there needs to be a balance of forces which make up the Qi, Yin (cold elements) and Yang (hot elements) (Lu 2004). Such a view is the basis of some alternative therapies such as acupuncture and differs greatly from the western biomedical approach to health. These alternative views have had an impact, medical domination is less than it was, people ask questions of their doctors and people are being more involved in decision-making about their care than ever before. The patient and the health care professionals are now seen as partners in care (NMC 2018; Oakley, Johl and Holber 2018; The King's Fund 2016).

Influences on Health

Until recently, there was a lack of acknowledgement of the many factors that influence our health. However, health is now seen as a balance between the body, the mind and the spirit and acknowledges the multiple factors which influence health. In order to become effective and efficient health promoters, it is essential to broaden our minds away from the narrowness of the biomedical model and understand the complex interplay of factors affecting health. Some factors which influence our health are constitutional and cannot be altered. Our genetics, our gender and our age are all such factors. However, many of the other influences we either impose on ourselves or are imposed on us by the society in which we live. We have more control over some factors than others; however, all factors are influenced by the way society is constructed (Dahlgren and Whitehead 1991, 2021). We may choose not to smoke tobacco, for instance, but this choice may be made harder for us if many of those within our social circle smoke. Some factors as individuals we have little choice over, for example, whether we become a victim of crime, although there are actions we can take to lessen this risk locking our doors, or being alert to fraudulent communications for instance. Table 1.1 gives a snapshot of some common influences on our health and illustrates the links between the choice the individual has, what that choice is dependent upon and what controls are exerted by society over that choice.

It can be seen from Table 1.1 that behavioural choices are complex decisions. It is important to see the bigger picture here as all too often individuals are held completely responsible for the way they live and the behaviour they exhibit. Unfortunately, individuals rarely have complete control over their environment and the choices which they make. Any person who has found the motivation to make a positive behaviour change ought to be commended as

Table 1.1 Examples of Health Influences and Variables Affecting These

Choice	Dependent on	Controlled or Influenced by
Drinking alcohol	Knowledge of safe alcohol limits Availability of alcohol to individuals Social acceptability amongst peers Income to purchase Access to drinking environment Addiction services for those wanting to limit intake	Health educators Licensing laws regarding premises, hours of sale, age limits for sale, responsible selling Alcohol manufactures Alcohol pricing Number of purchasing outlets Health policy and funding
Cycling	Income to purchase equipment Individual ability to ride Individual ability to store equipment Individual motivation and enjoyment Time available Provision of safe environment	Cycling organisations, lobbying groups Local authorities, transport and leisure departments, highways agency Manufacturers of equipment Cycle retailers Workplace cycle schemes Health educators
Eating a healthy diet	Knowledge of what constitutes a healthy diet Individual and family motivation Income to purchase healthy food Cooking skills Cooking and eating facilities	Food standards agency Farmers and food producers Food manufacturers and retail agreements. Labelling guidelines Food pricing
Level of educational attainment	Intellectual ability and motivation Supportive family and cultural environment Income to purchase equipment, e.g. computers and textbooks Good quality educational environment Good teachers Cost of education to individual Qualification infrastructure, exam boards, awarding bodies	Education acts – age and level of compulsory education by law. Level of Government and Local Authority funding for buildings and learning resources Quality of teacher training Educational watchdogs and quality control organisations
Smoking cannabis	Access to sales network for drug Income to purchase Social acceptability amongst peers Addiction services for those wanting to quit Education and prevention services	Drug laws Police Health educators Health policy and funding
Regular social contact	Access to supportive social circle Transport to meeting places Individual motivation and skills Income to purchase activities Variety of activities available	Public and private transport infrastructure and funding Regulation of safe activities Groups of individuals with particular interests

they are battling against the limitations that society places on them. Moreover, society also puts laws, guidelines, agreements and funding in place to aid positive health behaviour change and to make healthy choices easier for individuals to make.

Activity

Think about the following factors and list the many ways each of these may negatively or positively affect health. A discussion of each of these factors is given at the end of this chapter.

- Unemployment
- The family we live with
- The political system of the country
- War
- The standard of housing in which we live
- Our level of self-confidence
- Air pollution

Perceptions of Health

Sociologists have studied the ways various sectors of society perceive health and have proposed theories to explain these. Some people adhere to the functionalist model or way of looking at health. They ignore their health needs and tend to seek help only when a condition interferes with what they consider to be their optimal level of function. They see themselves as healthy as long as they can perform their perceived roles and responsibilities in the workplace or in the home (Yang, Bekemeier and Choi 2018). Even if they are in pain or develop a rash or lose a certain degree of mobility, for example, as long as they can perform the necessary tasks in their daily lives, they consider themselves to be healthy. This limited expectation of what constitutes health is a common one, especially amongst working class societies who generally have less expectations of good health than do the affluent sectors of the population (Barry and Yull 2021). Different genders also view health differently. Men are much more likely to view their body as a machine which occasionally breaks down and needs to be fixed. Men are generally less likely to discuss symptoms with other men and are also less likely to seek help and can often therefore leave problems until they have deteriorated to a dangerous degree (Novak et al. 2019). This attitude is a serious one as from birth to the age of 75 years male mortality significantly outstrips that of female mortality (Worldbank.org 2022). It has been argued that this reluctance by men to access health care or indeed adopt preventative health measures is the result of the perceived need by men to conform to a masculine identity, one which values strength and decries weakness and ill health as a feminine indulgence (Addis and Mahalik 2003; Arber and Cooper 2000; Smith, Mouzon and Elliott 2018). There are numerous examples of men waiting many months or years suspecting that various symptoms they are experiencing may be indicative of some disease but failing to present for investigation (Institute of Cancer Research [ICR] 2009). In 2009, research by Cancer Research UK found that men were 40% more likely to die of cancer than women (Cohen 2009). This hesitancy to seek treatment coupled with more risk-taking activities, for example, higher alcohol and smoking rates, has been traditionally cited as the reason why male cancer rates are generally higher than women's. However, recent years have seen more research into this issue and it is becoming clear that this is not the only story. Scientists have shown that women tend to have more protection than men because of their genetic make-up, especially the fact that women have two X chromosomes which contain tumour suppressors (Odonnell 2017). This, coupled to the possible role of oestrogen, appears to give women a higher cancer survival rate (Kim et al. 2018), but it is a multifactorial and complex picture. Women tend to define health more in terms of social relationships than men do; they tend to discuss symptoms more with each other and are more likely to present to health care professionals than men are when they do have a problem (Barry and Yull 2021). Statistics show that between the age of 16 and 60 men use health care services far less than women do (Wang et al. 2013). This may be the result of more emotional openness, but also women are generally brought into contact with health care services much more than the average man. Young women tend to seek contraceptive services; they may become pregnant and then later they access health care with their children. In middle age, symptoms associated with the menopause may also make them seek help. This makes the average woman probably much more familiar with health care provision than the average man, who, provided that he stays well, may not access health care until late middle age. Given this circumstance, it is not surprising that he is reluctant to enter a system about which he has no knowledge and also has to disclose intensely personal aspects of himself (Novak et al. 2019). Younger people are more likely to see health as an infinite resource. They value the physical fitness, strength and vitality they possess and cannot envisage ever being without this. This leads to more risk-taking behaviour in the 12–24 years age groups than in older people. Young adults can also be at a disadvantage through low income and poor housing and also start unhealthy behaviour such as smoking, alcohol and drug use which have ramifications for the future (Hagell et al. 2018; Sanci, Webb, and Hocking 2018). People in the middle age group have a more rounded notion of health which incorporates a feeling of mental and social well-being as well as physical functioning. The middle-aged, especially the more affluent and those educated to a degree level and above, are likely to take preventative health steps in their middle years (BMJ.com 2020; Halcomb et al. 2021). Older people have less expectations of good health, and they generally expect to have aches and pains and have less physical prowess than when they were younger. However, they value their ability to live independent lives and perform common tasks and daily routines and this becomes their benchmark for health. There seems to be a reluctance to be seen as being ill and a strong motivation towards feeling and being seen as healthy (Tkatch et al. 2017; Warmoth et al. 2015). The obvious difficulty is that as health means so many different things to different people, it is quite a task to be able to positively influence health, to promote good health.

Perceptions of Illness

The above discussion raises the question that if there are differing opinions to what constitutes health. it is logical that there is the same issue with what constitutes ill health. Often, ill health is perceived by the individual as something that differs from the norm. In the 1980s, the members of a tribe in South America were discovered to have a disfiguring skin condition. The condition had become so widespread within the population that it was considered a normal or healthy state. So distorted was this perception that the few individuals free of the infection were considered abhorrent and were refused the right to marry and pass on their immunity to succeeding generations (Zola 1983). However, it isn't just in primitive societies that such situations occur; in western societies ill health is also socially constructed to some extent. Societal acceptability plays a role in defining ill health. In the Victorian era, women who transgressed societal norms and had affairs and illegitimate offspring ran the risk of being diagnosed insane and committed to asylums. In developed nations, people who state that they can hear voices are likely to receive a diagnosis of schizophrenia and receive medication to block these. In primitive societies, such a person may be revered as being able to speak to the spirit world and declared a highly respected Shaman (Versola-Russo 2005). Attitude to disability is an excellent example of how things have changed. Children with disabilities were until recently placed in special schools and considered to have no future in contributing positively to society; rather, they would need care for the rest of their lives, by the state and their families. During the last 40 years or so, attitudes have changed. The aim is to present a positive view of disability, a social model rather than a medical model. In the social model, the emphasis is on how society needs to change in order for the people with disabilities to be integrated into and contribute to society, whereas the medical model focused on the problems the disabled person had and how to change or fix them so that they fitted into society as it is (Office of Disability Issues [ODI] 2012; UK Gov n.d.). The result has largely been a sea change in attitudes to disability and the people with disabilities have commanded much more respect and greater expectations are placed on them. The Paralympic Games have done much to increase respect for disabled athletes, especially those with physical impairments. However, it needs to be remembered that these are the elite, not the norm. In 2020 in the UK, only 52% of disabled people were in employment compared to 82% of the non-disabled population, and amongst those on the Autistic Spectrum only 22% were in employment (Parliament UK 2021). As unemployment or underemployment is linked to poverty (UN 2018), this is a highly significant and fundamental cause of inequality worldwide (Health Equity Organisation 2020).

What Is Public Health?

Definitions of Public Health

The most well-recognised definition of public health is perhaps the following: '*The science and art of preventing disease, prolonging life and promoting health through the organised efforts and informed choices of society, organisations, public and private, communities and individuals*' (Winslow 1920). Although given in the 1920s, the definition stands the test of time. Public health is not only about reducing mortality rates, but also about improving the quality of life. This definition also introduces the idea that promoting health is everyone's responsibility. Individuals make choices which affect health. Also, as we have seen, the way society acts and is constructed also affects health. Within this, governments, both national and local, play a part, as do health services, employers, community groups, families, etc. Winslow also acknowledges in the phrase 'science and art', that it is not solely medical discoveries that contribute to good health, important though these are, but also the less defined factors that contribute to the way that we feel. Our social relationships, the environment that we live in and our sense of purpose may be some of the factors he considered to be the arts of public health.

The Work of Public Health

Perhaps, it is also useful to discuss the principles of public health practice. Healthworks, a forum that styles itself as being made up of the world's best thinkers in health care, has stated the following principles as being essential to public health (UK Public Health Network 2022):

- To improve the health and well-being of populations, communities, families and individuals
- To prevent disease and minimise its consequences
- To prolong valued life
- To reduce inequalities in health

These are in general agreement with Winslow. The only difference is the inclusion of the principle to reduce inequalities in health. This has become a fundamental goal in public health in recent decades and will be discussed in more depth in the following chapter. Added to this should also be health surveillance. This work is the collecting of data about the prevalence and incidence of disease and behavioural factors which lead to disease. Statistics in the UK are generally collated by the Office of National Statistics, the UK Health Security Agency and the NHS, but health professionals, charities, local government and researchers all contribute to this essential gathering of information, without which it would be impossible to know the extent of problems, the trend of those problems and indeed if interventions are proving to be effective.

Health Promotion

Health promotion is an important arm of public health practice and has been defined as '*the process of enabling individuals and communities to increase control over the determinants of health and thereby improve their health*' (WHO 1986). Health promotion as a defined practice is relatively new in comparison to public health, only establishing itself towards the end of the 20th century. A series of health promotion charters have been created, stating the guiding principles of health promotion, perhaps the most significant being the Ottawa Charter of 1986. Key points in this charter were as follows:

- Creating healthy public policy so that laws passed, taxation levied and guidelines and standards set by national and local governments should take account of and strive to improve health.
- Creating supportive environments to improve health so that people live in safe and satisfying environments which protect natural resources.
- Strengthen community action by encouraging people to engage in health both for their community and themselves.
- Develop the personal skills of individuals so that they will have the information and skills to make informed decisions about their health and cope with health issues they face.
- Reorientation of health services from illness services to services which focus more on the prevention of disease and the promotion of well-being (WHO 1986).

Health education, informing and raising awareness of health issues, forms part of health promotion and is a vital first step in promoting health. It is essential for people to know the risks of certain behaviours before they can be expected to change this behaviour (Health Literacy UK 2015). At first sight, the principles of health promotion don't seem too different from those of public health and there is certainly overlap if not a little rivalry. The important thing is not to get carried away by semantics.

Figure 1.1 probably best explains how the different strands of public health work together.

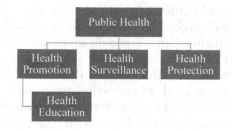

Figure 1.1 The Work of Public Health

The Growth and Changing Nature of Public Health

Throughout history, people have sought ways to limit ill health and the spread of disease. During the plague, people carried around oranges, studded with pungent spices such as cloves in them, thinking that in warding away the smell of disease, the disease itself would be kept at bay. This is because, until the 19th century, causes of disease and methods of transmission were largely unknown. A common belief was the miasma theory which had dominated for centuries and was based on the notion that contaminated air was responsible for spreading disease (Patwardhan, Mutalik and Tillu 2015). This theory was superseded by germ theory once microorganisms were proved to be responsible for infectious disease. The birth of the modern public health movement arose out of this discovery and the need to combat the appalling number of deaths caused by infection. Before the days of antibiotics, which were not in common usage until after the Second World War, public health measures undertaken focused on cleanliness, better housing with less overcrowding, clean water supply and sewage and better nutrition, all of which combined contributed to the dramatic drop in deaths caused by infectious disease (Environmental Health Perspectives 2019; Rosen 2015). In England and Wales in 1840, there were 70 deaths from measles per each 100,000 of the population (Office of National Statistics [ONS] 1997), whereas in 2007 only one child died from measles in the whole of the UK (Health Protection Agency 2012). The trend is the same for all the common childhood diseases. Medical advances had played their part, widespread vaccination for smallpox was established in the Victorian period and antiseptics were created and used widely. However, as vaccination for most childhood illnesses and other diseases such as tuberculosis was not available until the later part of the 20th century, it is the improved living conditions aided by widespread improvement in standard of living over this period that should take the credit for this change (Baggott 2010; Rosen 2015). Unfortunately, the world is not free of infectious disease and the overuse of antibiotics has caused microbial resistance. The COVID-19 pandemic had accounted for more than 5.5 million deaths worldwide by January 2022, with the cases still rising (Johns Hopkins Coronavirus Resource Center 2022). Besides causing widespread deaths and disability, it caused massive global economic and social disruption, detrimentally impacting livelihoods and the food supply (WHO 2020). COVID-19 is spread by aerosol particles that people breathe in and so people living in overcrowded accommodation are more at risk. Many other infectious diseases are caused by poor water supply and sanitation and it is important to stress that improvement in living conditions is an essential first step to combat infectious disease. Developed nations have numerous regulations to govern the standards of housing, water supply, food safety and sanitation which we take for granted. Such standards are not universal in the developing world and many preventable deaths still occur (Healthpovertyaction.org 2018; Hood 2005). The WHO states that diarrhoeal diseases are the second most common cause of death in under five-year-olds. This is a result of poor hygiene around bottle feeding. If infants were exclusively breastfed for their first six months of life, one million children's lives would be saved (WHO 2017). Tuberculosis (TB), measles and malaria remain endemic especially in the developing world with 1.5 million dying of TB in 2018 (Foster 2020). In the same year, it was estimated that 26 million people were living with HIV in sub-Saharan Africa (WHO Regional Office for Africa 2018). Relatively cheap and cost-effective methods of prevention are available to address these specific health issues, such as the provision of insecticide-treated mosquito nets to combat malaria, which has been estimated to reduce malaria deaths in the under five-year-olds by 63% (Medical Research Council 2012). Distribution of free condoms to prevent the spread of HIV is also an important preventative measure, although agencies working in this field realise that hand in hand with this is the work that goes on facilitating discussions around sexual health and safe sex within communities which helps challenge current attitudes and behaviour (Bom et al. 2019). In addition, as developing countries join the economic revolution and sections of the society become more affluent, individuals adopt the unhealthy habits of western nations. Smoking and obesity levels increase and with them the burden of chronic diseases such as diabetes and cardiovascular disease prevalent in the developed world. The developing world is therefore said to suffer from a dual burden of disease, that of infectious disease because of poverty and that of chronic disease as the result of affluence (Kushitor and Boatemaa 2018; Thelancet.com 2019).

Modern-Day Public Health Roles in the UK

Within developed nations, it is the burden of chronic disease which now accounts for much of the focus of the public health movement. In 2020, the Chief Medical Officer for England's Annual Report showed that on an average people in the UK spend around 20% of their lifespan in ill health (Chief Medical Officer 2020). As people grow older, the number of chronic conditions that people live with multiplies. The most common of these diseases are musculoskeletal problems, such as chronic back pain, or arthritis and heart and circulatory problems, such as previous heart attacks or high blood pressure. Diabetes is also common (CMO 2020). Behavioural factors play a large part in the acquisition of such diseases; for instance, an unhealthy diet and obesity lead to coronary heart disease and diabetes and also puts excess weight and therefore stress on joints leading to osteoarthritis. Risk factors will be discussed in more depth in the following chapter, but it is the limiting of these risk factors by providing information and supporting people through behavioural change that forms much of the work of health promoters working in public health. In addition to combating the growth of chronic diseases and reducing health inequalities, the public health workforce has a responsibility to tackle acute problems, such as an outbreak of salmonella or meningitis, or on a more global level to work with other nations to combat climate change and prevent pandemics such as influenza and COVID-19 and to take measures to prevent spread. The public health workforce also responds to emergencies. A common problem in recent years in the UK has been flooding. Emergency plans ensure that all services work together to provide clean drinking water when supplies have been disrupted and arrange emergency shelters for those affected (Institute of Health Promotion and Education 2022).

Who Is Involved in Public Health?

We have already discussed that health is a very diverse topic with many influences which come under the remit of most of society in one way or the other. To get a snapshot of those workers who see themselves as directly influencing public health and are probably the

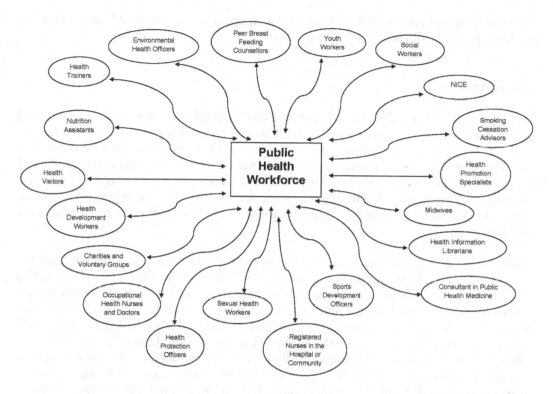

Figure 1.2 The Public Health Workforce

readers of this text (see Figure 1.2). The number of workers, both paid and unpaid who see public health as part of their role, is expanding year after year. In England, responsibility for health prevention and promotion and the wider determinants of health comes under the Office for Health Improvement and Disparities (OHID), part of the Department of Health and Social Care. Local authorities are then charged with commissioning public health services and leading on local health improvement and prevention. The National Health Service, meanwhile, is focused very much on the diagnosis and treatment of existing diseases and is less well equipped to address the multiple factors which influence health. Decisions regarding priorities and the funding of projects are made at the local authorities' Health and Well Being boards, comprising public health services, local counsellors, members of the public, GPs and hospital and community health care representatives (Gov.UK 2021). Below this national and local commissioning level are a wide range of grassroots workers who put into action policies decided at the national or local government level (Department of Health 2012). Some workers such as health promotion specialists may work with neighbourhoods to help them set their own priorities and work on specific projects, a toy library or a community garden, for instance. Registered nurses will work more 1-1 with their patients to provide information and support them with self-care and behaviour change (NMC 2018). Youth workers provide positive role models, activities and an enjoyable and safe environment for young people, thus enhancing physical and mental health. Community nutrition assistants work in communities and schools to discuss ways of eating healthily and teach cooking skills. Then there is the workforce which is influenced by government priorities, and also sets its own agenda, charities such as MIND for mental health and Help the Aged for older people. Occupational health physicians and nurses are employed by companies and organisations to ensure that the working environment is safe and health promoting. All in all, the public health workforce is vast.

Activity Answers

Unemployment: Limited income gives limited choices in all areas of life and there is a need to prioritise essentials and cheap alternatives. This affects people's physical health, for example, poor diet and lack of access to structured leisure opportunities. Also, their mental health, with a greater risk of social isolation, lack of sense of purpose, decreased self-worth and self-confidence, lack of motivation and depression. These are just a few examples of the ways that unemployment affects health. It has a major detrimental effect on health and causes an increase in ill health and premature death (Marmot 2015; Norström et al. 2019; Wilkinson and Marmot 2003).

Family: Family attitudes and behaviour influence family members' own attitudes and behaviour, parents influence children and partners influence each other (Davis-Kean 2005; Robards et al., 2012). With regard to health, this may be a positive or negative influence. A child of a smoker is more likely to start smoking, often obtaining their early cigarettes from their parents (Action on Smoking and Health 2019). A household who values educational attainment is likely to pass on that value to their offspring (Social Market Foundation 2020). Family responsibilities are also important. By far the greatest degree of caring happens informally within families, often older people caring for partners or middle-aged children caring for parents. This can have a significant effect on the health of the carers themselves. It is estimated that in the UK one in eight adults are carers, many of whom juggle work and caring, or if unable to do so, give up work because of the need to care for someone. Eighty percent of carers reported that caring had left them socially isolated and over 60% said that caring had contributed to physical or mental health problems (CarersUK.org 2021). Caring for disabled children or those suffering from serious illness also puts a tremendous strain on family members and relationships. Research has shown that parents with disabled children have higher levels of stress and lower levels of well-being than parents with non-disabled children (Brook 2011; Masefield et al. 2020). Domestic relationships, if strong and supportive, have a significant positive influence on health; conversely, unhappy relationships or those containing domestic violence have the opposite effect (Robards et al. 2012). Research has shown that partners in unfulfilling, unsatisfactory relationships are at increased risk of cardiovascular disease and chronic pain (McWilliams and Bailey 2010; Robles, Slatcher and Trombello et al. 2014). Whatever the issue, the problems of family members have ramifications for all those in the family. However, the opposite is true – supportive families increase the health status of those in them. Adults benefit from supportive partnerships and children growing up in supportive homes have greater self-confidence to go forward into adult life and meet its challenges (The Health Foundation 2018).

The Political System of the Country: Politics is closely bound to health care and public health policy. In the UK, the health service is a nationalised body run by the government. As the NHS is funded by taxation, it is important for the government of the day to show the electorate that it provides value for money and effective practice. Health is a very emotive subject and populations have strong views about priorities and what should be available and what should be paid for privately. The problem is, there are obviously differences in opinions and the running of health services is often seen as a political football with different political parties using health care to score points against the opposition (Rimmer and Iacobucci 2019). The watchword is reform. The term is synonymous with change, but continuous change is unsettling and costs money in itself. Each restructuring is said to cost at least two years of progress in health care provision (Edwards 2011). This drive to change is true around the world, not just in the UK health care system. In stable political systems, such as operating in the developed world, health care systems despite differences in operation are largely available to the majority of the population of the country. However, in poorer developing nations, provision, especially for the poorest, is by no means certain. Public health or health promotion programmes are often seen as the Cinderella end of provision, with the largest pots of funding going to secondary (hospital) treatment and care rather than preventative services.

War: War is of course closely linked to the political system of the country. At first sight, it may seem obvious how war affects the health of a nation. People will get killed and maimed. There are also many indirect effects of war on an individual's health. The death of loved ones causes severe emotional trauma. It can have a significant impact on the income of the family and family members may be required to take on additional responsibilities. Wars shatter communities, houses are destroyed and people are displaced (Wheeler 2020). Also, in war, the nations' resources are redirected to support the war effort. This may mean a lack of funding for other things, developments in health care for instance. Infrastructure, including roads and railways, may be destroyed, sanitation and water supply disrupted, and education suffers, with schools often closing due to the perceived danger. Manufacturing output may boom which leads to a temporary increase in employment, but generally war is very bad news for health (Sidal and Levy 2008).

Housing Standards: In the developed world, the standard of housing is regulated and minimum standards have to be in place. This is not true of much of the developing world where the poorest of the population often live in appalling conditions without adequate water supply, correct sanitation, security and space. Poor housing in such regions leads to large prevalence of infectious disease and injury (WHO 2022). However, western nations cannot be complacent as poor housing still affects the health of those in developed countries. Overcrowding assists the spread of disease, poor insulation and inefficient heating contribute to fuel poverty and winter deaths and poor layout and inadequate safety equipment lead to accidental injury and deaths in fires. Lack of personal space affects mental health and also children's educational attainment (Habitat for Humanity 2022). Good planning can address these issues. Good ventilation, hardwood flooring and damp-free homes cut down the incidence and severity of asthma. Planned community building which incorporates open spaces, cycle and walking routes, shops and public facilities such as libraries and leisure centres promotes social cohesion and lessens crime (Housing Matters 2017).

Levels of Self-Confidence: Our level of self-confidence is bound up strongly with our self-efficacy, the belief that we can achieve something. This is especially relevant when discussing behaviour change, as we need to believe that we can achieve change before we embark on it. This is a key tenet of the health belief model which will be discussed in more detail later (Rosenstock, Strecher and Becker 1988). Self-confidence can also contribute to assertiveness. Those with self-confidence are more likely to seek out useful information from others, join support groups, speak their mind and be more proactive, all of which lead to less social isolation and more engagement in society. They are more likely to have less anxiety and depression and better mental health (MacInnes 2006; Nguyen et al. 2019).

Air Pollution: The WHO now classes air pollution on par with smoking as a major cause of diseases and disability (WHO 2021). Air pollution is a significant causal factor in respiratory diseases, cancer, coronary heart disease and stroke, and there are also links between air pollution and dementia, diabetes, obesity and inflammatory disease (European Environment Agency 2021). Those most at risk are children, older people and those with chronic diseases. Fine particulate matter from coal power stations, fires and vehicle exhausts can bypass defences in our nose and respiratory passages, thereby entering our lungs and from there into our bloodstream (European Environment Agency 2021). The WHO recently updated their guidelines for maximum levels of various pollutants both for indoor and outdoor settings (WHO 2021). Motor vehicle transport releases carbon dioxide, sulphur dioxide and nitrogen dioxide. Removing older vehicles, increasing the use of vehicles with stop-start technology to prevent idling, switching to electric vehicles and obviously using our cars less will all help to reduce this major pollutant as well as help to reduce climate change.

Key Messages

- Health is socially constructed and people hold differing views on what it is to be healthy.
- Virtually everything in society affects our health to a greater or lesser extent.
- The developed world has more resources to control infectious disease and much of the work of public health now concentrates on limiting chronic diseases such as cardiovascular disease, diabetes and cancer.
- The developing world has both a high incidence of infectious disease and an increasing amount of chronic disease.
- Public health is made up of different aspects: Health Promotion, Health Education, Health Surveillance and Health Protection.
- Many people are involved in public health either directly or indirectly, whether they work for local authorities or the NHS and charitable institutions or private organisations.

References

Action on Smoking and Health. (2019). *Young people and smoking factsheet* [online]. Available at: https://ash.org.uk/information-and-resources/fact-sheets/young-people-and-smoking/
Addis, M.E. and Mahalik, J.R. (2003). Men, masculinity, and the contexts of help seeking. *American Psychologist*, 58, pp. 5–14.
Antonovsky, A. (1979). *Health, stress and coping*. San Francisco, CA: Jossey-Bass.
Antonovsky, A. (1996). The salutogenic model as a theory to guide health promotion. *Health Promotion International*, 11, pp. 11–18.
Arber, S. and Cooper, H. (2000). Gender and inequalities in health across the lifecourse, in Annandale, E and Hunt, K (eds.) *Gender inequalities in health*. Buckingham Open University Press. pp. 625–647.
Baggott, R. (2010). *Public health policy and politics*. 2nd ed. Basingstoke: Palgrave Macmillan.
Barry, A.M. and Yull, C. (2021). *Understanding the sociology of health*. 4th ed. Peterborough: SAGE.
Bircher, J. (2005). Towards a dynamic definition of health and disease. *Medical. Health Care Philosophy*, 8, pp. 335–341.
Bmj.com. (2015). *Too much medicine* [online]. Available at: https://www.bmj.com/too-much-medicine

Bmj.com. (2020). *Healthy habits in middle age linked to longer life free from disease* [online]. Available at: https://www.bmj.com/company/newsroom/healthy-habits-in-middle-age-linked-to-longer-life-free-from-disease/

Bom, R.J.M., van der Linden, K., Matser, A., Poulin, N., Schim van der Loeff, M.F., Bakker, B.H.W. and van Boven, T.F. (2019). The effects of free condom distribution on HIV and other sexually transmitted infections in men who have sex with men. *BMC Infectious Diseases* [online], 19(1). Available at: https://bmcinfectdis.biomedcentral.com/articles/10.1186/s12879-019-3839-0#:~:text=of%20 the%20intervention.-,Conclusions,chlamydia%2C%20gonorrhoea%2C%20and%20syphilis

Brook, A. (2011). Parenting under pressure and the SEN parent. *Special Educational Needs Magazine*. Available at: http://www.senmagazine.co.uk/articles/404-parenting-under-pressure-stress-and-the-sen-parent.html

Carersuk.org. (2021). *Facts and figures - Carers UK* [online]. Available at: https://www.carersuk.org/ news-and-campaigns/press-releases/facts-and-figures

Chief Medical Officer's Annual Report. (2020). *Health trends and variation in England* [online]. Available at: https://assets.publishing.service.gov.uk/government/uploads/system/uploads/attachment_ data/file/945929/Chief_Medical_Officer_s_annual_report_2020_-_health_trends_and_variation_ in_England.pdf

Cohen, D. (2009). Men need primary care at work, debate hears. *British Medical Journal*, 338, p. b2471.

Conrad, P. and Barker, K. (2010). The social construction of illness: Key insights and policy implications. *Journal of Health and Social Behavior*, 51, pp. 67–79.

Dahlgren, G. and Whitehead, M. (1991). *Policies and strategies to promote social equity in health*. Stockholm. Sweden: Institute for Futures Studies.

Dahlgren, G. and Whitehead, M. (2021). The Dahlgren-Whitehead model of health determinants: 30 years on and still chasing rainbows. *Public Health* [online], 199, pp. 20–24. Available at: https:// www.sciencedirect.com/science/article/pii/S003335062100336X

Davis-Kean, P.E. (2005). The influence of parent education and family income on child achievement: The indirect role of parental expectations and the home environment. *Journal of Family Psychology*, 19, pp. 294–304.

Department of Health. (2012). *The new public health role of local authorities* [online]. Available at: https://assets.publishing.service.gov.uk/government/uploads/system/uploads/attachment_data/ file/213009/Public-health-role-of-local-authorities-factsheet.pdf

Edwards, N. (2011). NHS reform is nothing new. *Health Service Journal*. Available at: http://m.hsj. co.uk/5031606.article

Engel, G.L. (1977). The need for a new medical model: A challenge for biomedicine. *Science*, 196(4286), pp. 129–136. https://doi.org/10.1126/science.847460

Environmental Health Perspectives. (2019). The relationship of housing and population health: A 30-year retrospective analysis. *Environmental Health Perspectives*, 117(4) [online]. Available at: https://ehp.niehs.nih.gov/doi/10.1289/ehp.0800086

European Environment Agency. (2021). *Air pollution: how it affects our health* [online]. Available at: https://www.eea.europa.eu/themes/air/health-impacts-of-air-pollution

Farre, A. and Rapley, T. (2017). The new old (and old new) medical model: Four decades navigating the biomedical and psychosocial understandings of health and illness. *Healthcare* [online], 5(4). Available at: https://pubmed.ncbi.nlm.nih.gov/29156540/

Foster, L. (2020). *What are some of the world's other infectious diseases – and how deadly are they?* [online], World Economic Forum. Available at: https://www.weforum.org/agenda/2020/04/covid-19-infectious-diseases-tuberculosis-measles-malaria/

GOV.UK. (2021). *Public health commissioning in the NHS: 2021 to 2022* [online]. Available at: https:// www.gov.uk/government/publications/public-health-commissioning-in-the-nhs-2021-to-2022

Green, J., Cross, R., Woodall, J. and Tones, K. (2019). *Health promotion: Planning and strategies*, 4th ed. London: Sage.

Habitat for Humanity. (2022). *How housing affects child development* [online]. Available at: https:// www.habitat.org/our-work/how-housing-affects-child-development

Hagell, A., Shah, R., People's Health, Y., Viner, R., Hargreaves, D., Varnes, L. and Heys, M. (2018). *The social determinants of young people's health. Identifying the key issues and assessing how young people are doing in the 2010s* [online]. Available at: https://www.health.org.uk/sites/default/files/The-social-determinants-of%20-young-peoples-health_0.pdf

Halcomb, E., Ashley, C., Middleton, R., Lucas, E., Robinson, K., Harvey, S., Charlton, K. and McInnes, S. (2021). Understanding perceptions of health, lifestyle risks and chronic disease in middle age. *Journal of Clinical Nursing* [online]. Available at: https://onlinelibrary.wiley.com/doi/abs/10.1111/jocn.15711

Health Equity Organisation. (2020). *Health equity in England: The Marmot review in England 10 years on* [online]. Available at: https://www.health.org.uk/sites/default/files/2020-03/Health%20Equity%20in%20England_The%20Marmot%20Review%2010%20Years%20On_executive%20summary_web.pdf

Health Literacy UK. (2015). *Why is health literacy important?* [online]. Available at: https://www.healthliteracy.org.uk/why-is-health-literacy-important

Healthpovertyaction.org. (2018). *Key facts: Poverty and poor health* [online]. Available at: https://www.healthpovertyaction.org/news-events/key-facts-poverty-and-poor-health/#:~:text=Overcrowded%20and%20poor%20living%20conditions, sanitation%20can%20also%20be%20fatal

Health Protection Agency. (2012). *Measles notification.* Available at: http://www.hpa.org.uk/web/HPAweb&HPAwebStandard/HPAweb_C/1195733835814

Henningsen, P. (2015). Still modern? Developing the biopsychosocial model for the 21st century. *Journal of Psychosomatic Research*, 79, pp. 362–363.

Hood, E. (2005). Dwelling disparities: How poor housing leads to poor health. *Environmental Health Perspectives*, 113(5), pp. A310–A317.

Housing Matters. (2017). *How housing quality affects child mental health* [online]. Available at: https://housingmatters.urban.org/articles/how-housing-quality-affects-child-mental-health

Institute of Cancer Research (ICR). (2009). *Everyman campaign.* Available at: http://everyman-campaign.org/

Institute of Health Promotion and Education. (2022). https://ihpe.org.uk/

Johns Hopkins Coronavirus Resource Center. (2022). *COVID-19 map - Johns Hopkins Coronavirus Resource Center* [online]. Available at: https://coronavirus.jhu.edu/map.html

Kim, H.-I., Lim, H. and Moon, A. (2018). Sex differences in cancer: Epidemiology, genetics and therapy. *Biomolecules & Therapeutics* [online], 26(4), pp. 335–342. Available at: https://www.ncbi.nlm.nih.gov/pmc/articles/PMC6029678/

Kushitor, M.K. and Boatemaa, S. (2018). *The double burden of disease and the challenge of health access: Evidence from access, bottlenecks, cost and equity facility survey in Ghana. PLOS ONE* [online], 13(3), p. e0194677. Available at: https://www.ncbi.nlm.nih.gov/pmc/articles/PMC5865721/

Lu, A.P. (2004). Theory of traditional Chinese medicine and therapeutic method of diseases. *World Journal of Gastroenterology* [online], 10(13), p. 1854. Available at: https://www.ncbi.nlm.nih.gov/pmc/articles/PMC4572216/

MacInnes, D.L. (2006). Self-esteem and self-acceptance: An examination into their relationship And their effect on psychological health. *Journal of Psychiatric Mental Health Nursing*, 13(5), pp. 483–489.

Marmot, M. (2015). *The health gap: The challenge of an unequal world.* London: Bloomsbury.

Masefield, S.C., Prady, S.L., Sheldon, T.A., Small, N., Jarvis, S. and Pickett, K.E. (2020). The caregiver health effects of caring for young children with developmental disabilities: A meta-analysis. *Maternal and Child Health Journal* [online], 24(5), pp. 561–574. Available at: https://www.ncbi.nlm.nih.gov/pmc/articles/PMC7170980

McWilliams, L.A. and Bailey, S.J. (2010). Associations between adult attachment ratings and health conditions: Evidence from the national comorbidity survey replication. *Health Psychology*, 29(4), pp. 446–453.

Medical Research Council. (2012). *Malaria mosquito nets.* Available at: http://www.mrc.ac.uk/Achievementsimpact/Storiesofimpact/Mosquitonets/index.htm

Mittelmark, M.B. and Bauer, G.F. (2022). The meanings of salutogenesis. *The handbook of salutogenesis* [online]. 2nd ed., pp. 7–13. Available at: https://www.ncbi.nlm.nih.gov/books/NBK435854/

National Health and Medical Research Council. (NHMRC). (1996). *Promoting the health of indigenous Australians. A review of infrastructure support for aboriginal and Torres Strait Islander health advancement.* Final report and recommendations. Canberra: NHMRC.

Nettleton, S. (1995). *The sociology of health and illness.* Cambridge: Polity.

Nguyen, D.T., Wright, E.P., Dedding, C., Pham, T.T. and Bunders, J. (2019). Low self-esteem and its association with anxiety, depression, and suicidal ideation in Vietnamese secondary school students: A cross-sectional study. *Frontiers in Psychiatry* [online], 10. Available at: https://www.frontiersin.org/articles/10.3389/fpsyt.2019.00698/full

Norström, F., Waenerlund, A.K., Lindholm, L., Nygren, R., Sahlén, K.G. and Brydsten, A. (2019). Does unemployment contribute to poorer health-related quality of life among Swedish adults? *BMC Public Health* [online], 19(1). Available at: https://bmcpublichealth.biomedcentral.com/articles/10.1186/s12889-019-6825-y

Novak, J.R., Peak, T., Gast, J. and Arnell, M. (2019). Associations between masculine norms and health-care utilization in highly religious, heterosexual men. *American Journal of Men's Health* [online], 13(3), 155798831985673. Available at: https://www.ncbi.nlm.nih.gov/pmc/articles/PMC6560804/

Nursing and Midwifery Council (NMC). (2018). *Future nurse: Standards of proficiency for registered nurses.* Available at: https://www.nmc.org.uk/globalassets/sitedocuments/standards-of-proficiency/nurses/future-nurse-proficiencies.pdf

Odonnell, J. (2017). Why is cancer more common in men? *Harvard Magazine* [online]. Available at: https://www.harvardmagazine.com/2017/03/why-is-cancer-more-common-in-men

O'Reilly, M. and Lester, J.N. (2016). Introduction: The social construction of normality and pathology. *The Palgrave Handbook of Adult Mental Health* [online], pp. 1–19. Available at: https://link.springer.com/chapter/10.1057/9781137496850_1

Oakley, C., Johl, R. and Holber, N. (2018). Holistic patient-centred care. *British Journal of Nursing*, 27(4) [online]. Available at: https://www.magonlinelibrary.com/doi/abs/10.12968/bjon.2018.27.4.S3 [accessed 23 March 2023].

Office of Disability Issues (ODI). (2012). *The social model of disability.* Available at: http://odi.dwp.gov.uk/about-the-odi/the-social-model.php

Office of National Statistics (ONS). (1997). *Recorded mortality in England and Wales.* London: ONS.

Parliament UK. (2018). *Disabled people in employment* [online]. Available at: https://researchbriefings.files.parliament.uk/documents/CBP-7540/CBP-7540.pdf

Patwardhan, B., Mutalik, G. and Tillu, G. (2015). Concepts of health and disease. *Integrative Approaches for Health* [online], pp. 53–78. Available at: https://www.sciencedirect.com/topics/medicine-and-dentistry/miasma-theory

Polhius, C.M.M., Vaandrager, L., Soedamah-Muthu, S.S. and Koelen, M.A. (2020). Salutogenic model of health to identify turning points and coping styles for eating practices in type 2 diabetes mellitus. *International Journal for Equity in Health* [online], 19(1). Available at: https://equityhealthj.biomedcentral.com/articles/10.1186/s12939-020-01194-4#:~:text=The%20Salutogenic%20Model%20is%20centred,and%20biochemical%20stressors%20%5B38%5D

Rimmer, A. and Iacobucci, G. (2019). NHS becomes political football as electioneering kicks off. *BMJ* [online], p. l6375. Available at: https://www.bmj.com/content/367/bmj.l6375

Robards, J., Evandrou, M., Falkingham, J. and Vlachantoni, A. (2012). Marital status, health and mortality. *Maturitas* [online], 73(4), pp. 295–299. Available at: https://www.ncbi.nlm.nih.gov/pmc/articles/PMC3635122/

Robles, T.F., Slatcher, R.B. and Trombello, J.M. (2014). Marital quality and health: A met-analytic review. *Psychological Bulletin*, 140(1), pp. 140–187.

Rosen, G. (2015). *A history of public health.* Revised ed. Baltimore: John Hopkins University Press.

Rosenstock, I.M., Strecher, V.J. and Becker, M.H. (1988). Social learning theory and the health belief model. *Health Education & Behavior*, 15(2), pp. 175–183.

Sanci, L., Webb, M. and Hocking, J. (2018). Risk taking behaviour in adolescents. *Australian Journal of General Practice* [online]. Available at: https://www1.racgp.org.au/ajgp/2018/december/risk-taking-behaviour-in-adolescents

Sidal, V.W. and Levy, B.S. (2008). The health impact of war. *International Journal of Injury Control and Safety Promotion*, 15(4), pp. 189–195.

Smith, D.T., Mouzon, D.M. and Elliott, M. (2018). Reviewing the assumptions about Men's mental health: An exploration of the gender binary. *American Journal of Men's Health* [online], 12(1), pp. 78–89. Available at: https://www.ncbi.nlm.nih.gov/pmc/articles/PMC5734543

Social Market Foundation. (2020). *Family matters: The role of parents in children's educational attainment – Social Market Foundation* [online]. Available at: https://www.smf.co.uk/publications/family-matters-role-parents-childrens-educational-attainment/

The Health Foundation. (2018). *How do our family, friends and community influence our health?* [online]. Available at: https://www.health.org.uk/infographic/how-do-our-family-friends-and-community-influence-our-health

The King's Fund. (2016). *Patients as partners* [online]. Available at: https://www.kingsfund.org.uk/publications/patients-partners

Thelancet.com. (2019). *The double burden of malnutrition* [online]. Available at: https://www.thelancet.com/series/double-burden-malnutrition#:~:text=The%20double%20burden%20of%20malnutrition%20is%20the%20coexistence%20of%20overnutrition,community%2C%20household%2C%20and%20individual

Tkatch, R., Musich, S., MacLeod, S., Kraemer, S., Hawkins, K., Wicker, E.R. and Armstrong, D.G. (2017). A qualitative study to examine older adults' perceptions of health: Keys to aging successfully. *Geriatric Nursing* [online], 38(6), pp. 485–490. Available at: https://pubmed.ncbi.nlm.nih.gov/28341064/

UK Gov. (n.d.). *Introduction to the social and medical models of disability* [online]. Available at: https://www.ombudsman.org.uk/sites/default/files/FDN-218144_Introduction_to_the_Social_and_Medical_Models_of_Disability.pdf

UK Public Health Network. (2022). https://ukpublichealthnetwork.org.uk/

United Nations (UN). (2018). Poverty eradication, inclusive growth focus of UN Social Development Commission's 2018 session - United Nations Sustainable Development [online]. United Nations Sustainable Development. Available at: https://www.un.org/sustainabledevelopment/blog/2018/01/poverty-eradication-inclusive-growth-focus-un-social-development-commissions-2018-session/

Ventres, W.B. and Frankel, R.M. (2021). Personalizing the BioPsychoSocial approach: "Add-ons" and "add-ins" in generalist practice. *Frontiers in Psychiatry* [online], 12. Available at: https://www.ncbi.nlm.nih.gov/pmc/articles/PMC8652412/

Versola-Russo, J.M. (2005). Cultural and demographic factors of schizophrenia. *International Journal of Psychosocial Rehabilitation*, 10(2), pp. 89–103.

Wade, D.T. and Halligan, P.W. (2004). Do biomedical models of illness make for good healthcare systems? *BMJ* [online], 329(7479), pp. 1398–1401. Available at: https://www.bmj.com/content/329/7479/1398.short

Wang, Y., Hunt, K., Nazareth, I., Freemantle, N. and Petersen, I. (2013). Do men consult less than women? An analysis of routinely collected UK general practice data. *BMJ Open* [online], 3(8), p. e003320. Available at: https://bmjopen.bmj.com/content/3/8/e003320

Warmoth, K., Tarrant, M., Abraham, C. and Lang, I.A. (2015). Older adults' perceptions of ageing and their health and functioning: A systematic review of observational studies. *Psychology, Health & Medicine* [online], 21(5), pp. 531–550. Available at: https://pubmed.ncbi.nlm.nih.gov/26527056/#:~:text=Many%20older%20people%20perceive%20ageing,or%20declining%20health%20and%20functioning.&text=Observational%20studies%20were%20included%20if,aged%2060%20years%20and%20older

Warwick-Booth, L. and Cross, R. (2018). *Global health studies: A social determinants perspective.* Cambridge: Polity.

Weston, W.W. (2005). Patient-centered medicine: A guide to the biopsychosocial model. *Family Systems and Health*, 23, pp. 387–392.

Wheeler, A.D.-C. (2020). *Health and harm: Protecting civilians and health.* Available at: https://article36.org/wp-content/uploads/2020/08/A36-protecting-health.pdf

Wilkinson, R. and Marmot, M. (Eds.) (2003). *Social determinants of health: The solid facts.* 2nd ed. Copenhagen: WHO Regional Office for Europe.

Winslow, C.E.A. (1920). The untilled fields of public health. *Science*, 51(1306), pp. 23–33.

Worldbank.org. (2022). *Life expectancy at birth, total (years) | Data* [online]. Available at: https://data.worldbank.org/indicator/SP.DYN.LE00.IN

World Health Organization (WHO). (1986). *Ottawa charter for health promotion.* Ottawa. WHO.

World Health Organization (WHO). (2017). *Diarrhoeal disease* [online]. Available at: https://www.who.int/news-room/fact-sheets/detail/diarrhoeal-disease [accessed 6 September 2021].

World Health Organization (WHO). (2020). *Impact of COVID-19 on people's livelihoods, their health and our food systems* [online]. Available at: https://www.who.int/news/item/13-10-2020-impact-of-covid-19-on-people's-livelihoods-their-health-and-our-food-systems [accessed 6 September 2021].

World Health Organization (WHO). (2021). *WHO global air quality guidelines: Particulate matter (PM2.5 and PM10), ozone, nitrogen dioxide, sulfur dioxide and carbon monoxide.* Available at: https://apps.who.int/iris/handle/10665/345329. License: CC BY-NC-SA 3.0 IGO.

World Health Organization (WHO). (2022). *Housing and health* [online]. Available at: https://www.euro.who.int/en/health-topics/environment-and-health/Housing-and-health [accessed 26 January 2022].

World Health Organization (WHO) Regional Office for Africa. (2018). *HIV/AIDS* [online]. Available at: https://www.afro.who.int/health-topics/hivaids [accessed 6 September 2021].

Yang, Y., Bekemeier, B. and Choi, J. (2018). A cultural and contextual analysis of health concepts and needs of women in a rural district of Nepal. *Global Health Promotion*, 25(1), pp. 15–22.

Zola, I.K. (1983). Missing pieces: *a chronicle of living with a disability.* Philadelphia. Temple University Press.

2 The Main Killers

Susan R. Thompson

Life Expectancy

A female child born in the UK in 2019 has an average life expectancy of 83 years and can expect to be healthy for around 66 years of that life. A male child born in the same year has a life expectancy of 79 years, with a healthy life of around 64 years (Office for National Statistics [ONS] 2020). This contrasts sharply with those countries of the world with the lowest life expectancy. In 2019 the Central African Republic had a life expectancy of only 53 years and Chad had a life expectancy of 54 years (World Bank 2021). We have become accustomed to life expectancy increasing year on year and perhaps have been complacent in expecting this trend to continue. However, even before the COVID-19 pandemic, increases in life expectancy had been slowing and were static in some nations including the United Kingdom in the years 2011–2018 (King's Fund 2021). Of all the major world economies, Japan tops the table for life expectancy, followed by Italy, France, Canada, UK and Germany in that order. Unfortunately, the USA comes in last at an average of just under 79 years compared with Japan's 84 years and the UK's 81.5 (Chief Medical Officer's Annual Report 2020). Prior to the COVID-19 epidemic, the World Health Organization (WHO) published data reflecting the leading causes of death and disability worldwide (see Table 2.1).

A close examination of both columns shows both diseases of affluence such as diabetes and diseases of poverty such as diarrhoeal disease. Causes of death obviously vary, depending on age as well as gender. In the under-fives, the leading cause of death are neonatal conditions, but in the developing world, it is diarrhoea, resulting from poor sanitation and living conditions. In England, in August 2021, the leading cause of death in adults was dementia and Alzheimer's disease, accounting for 11% of all deaths. Ischaemic heart disease (IHD) came second while COVID-19 came third at 6%. In 2020, the leading cause of deaths in adults in England and Wales had been COVID-19 at 12% of all deaths (ONS 2021b). The pandemic has obviously had a significant impact on mortality statistics worldwide and at this point its lasting legacy is unknown, although it appears that it will be with us for some considerable time in one form or another. It remains to be seen how much vaccination and treatments will be able to combat variants that will inevitably emerge.

Accidents are the primary cause of deaths in young adults who are classed as those under the age of 44. In the USA, in 2019, almost half of these deaths were motor vehicle related, and the remaining deaths were due to accidental poisoning, mainly drug overdoses, a trend that has been rising steadily since the early 2000s. Suicide is unfortunately the second major cause of death in young adults in both the USA and the UK after accidental injury (Centers

DOI: 10.4324/9781003411321-2

Table 2.1 The Most Common Causes of Death and Disability Worldwide 2019 (WHO 2021a)

Top Ten Global Causes of Death in 2019	Top Ten Global Causes of Disability Adjusted Life Years (DALYs) in 2019
Ischaemic heart disease	Neonatal conditions
Stroke	Ischaemic heart disease
Chronic obstructive pulmonary disease	Stroke
Lower respiratory infections	Lower respiratory infections
Neonatal conditions	Diarrhoeal diseases
Trachea, bronchus, lung cancers	Road injury
Alzheimer's disease and other dementias	Chronic obstructive pulmonary disease
Diarrhoeal diseases	Diabetes mellitus
Diabetes mellitus	Tuberculosis
Kidney diseases	Congenital anomalies

for Disease Control and Prevention 2021; ONS 2020), but it is wrong to assume that suicide is a problem purely associated with more affluent countries. The WHO estimates that suicide is a major issue worldwide, and in those nations where suicide is still illegal, it is grossly underreported (WHO 2021b). Amongst older adults, vascular dementia and Alzheimer's disease were reported as the leading cause of death in the UK in 2018, followed by IHD and cancer (ONS 2020). The most common forms of cancer in the UK are breast, prostate, lung and bowel (Cancerdata 2023). As you can see in Table 2.1, the leading cause of death and disability worldwide remains ischaemic heart disease and stroke. This was a familiar pattern in more developed countries until medical advances in medication and surgical procedures enabled people with IHD to live longer lives. Unfortunately, people living in developing countries do not always have access to these advanced treatments, hence the continued dominant prevalence of IHD.

Healthy Life Expectancy

Along with life expectancy (LE), it is also important to consider healthy life expectancy (HLE). This is the period of an individual's life which he or she can expect to live in good health. HLE is reached when an individual starts getting affected by a disability or long-term condition which directly affects their health status and forces them to get into contact with health and social care services on a regular basis, rather than for a one-off acute episode. We also talk about the 'window of need'. This is the period between acquiring a condition which requires long-term healthcare and death. The aim is to reduce that window so that people can be healthy for a longer part of their lives. Trends show that although life expectancy is gradually increasing, in Western societies this is not necessarily mirrored by advances in healthy life expectancy and that although we are living longer, we are not necessarily spending that time in good health (All Party Parliamentary Group for Longevity 2021). Women, although generally living longer than men, have an equivalent HLE and, consequently, spend a greater proportion of their life affected by poor health (ONS 2022) (see Table 2.2). Older people were adversely affected by the COVID-19 pandemic, not just from higher risk of death, but also from restrictions in their daily lives lived in a climate of fear. Perhaps worse affected were those living in care homes, especially those with a diagnosis of dementia or Alzheimer's disease. Lockdowns caused a marked decrease in social contact of patients with dementia, which significantly worsened their condition. Forty-six percent of people with this diagnosis reported a negative impact on their mental health

Table 2.2 Healthy Life Expectancy in the UK 2014–2016 and 2017–2019. ONS (2022) Health and Life Expectancies

	Years 2014–2016		Years 2017–2019	
	Life Expectancy	Healthy Life Expectancy	Life Expectancy	Healthy Life Expectancy
Males	78	62	79	62
Females	83	64	84	63

while 82% reported deteriorating symptoms due to lack of social contact during this time (Alzheimer's Society UK 2020).

HLE, like LE, is also impacted by deprivation, with those living in more deprived circumstances having a lower HLE than those living more affluently (ONS 2022).

Non-Modifiable Risk Factors

Increasing age, genetics, ethnic background and gender all play a part in putting us under the risk of contracting specific diseases. Such factors are termed non-modifiable as there is little we can do to influence these. Individuals are more at risk of cardiovascular disease (CVD) as they age, men are more prone than women (although after the menopause women's risk equals that of men), and if a close male family member had a heart attack before the age of 55 or if a close female family member had one before the age of 65, other close family members are at increased risk. A close family member is defined as a parent or sibling (American Heart Association 2021; British Heart Foundation [BHF] 2021). Physicians, family doctors and nurses use risk assessment tools to gauge an individual's likelihood to develop CVD, based on the risk factors that they exhibit (Qrisk.org. 2018). The factors considered are multiple and include medical history, age, gender, smoking habit, systolic blood pressure, the ratio of total cholesterol to HDL/LDL cholesterol and body mass index. A score for that individual is calculated which equates to a percentage risk he or she has of developing CVD within the next ten-year period. When this percentage is 20% or above in individuals yet to show symptoms of CVD, lifestyle advice and clinical treatment, such as cholesterol lowering statins and anti-hypertensive medication, is commenced to reduce this risk (Qrisk.org. 2018). These interventions are also commenced with people who have diabetes and those with an existing diagnosis of CVD (those with angina for instance).

COVID-19

COVID-19 obviously influenced life expectancy during the period of the pandemic, reducing life expectancy in the UK, Spain, Portugal, France and Poland (Limb 2021). Increasing age is the most significant risk factor of death from COVID-19, with the average age at death in England and Wales in 2020 being 80 years (ONS 2021a). Diabetes has been found to be the most significant long-term condition associated with death from COVID-19; 23.0% of people who died of COVID-19 in England and Wales in the first six months of 2021 were also diabetics (Diabetes UK 2021). Dementia and Alzheimer's disease were also significant risk factors for death, but 13% of people who died of COVID-19 within this period had no long-term condition at all (ONS 2021b).

Critical thinking

Take some time to research and consider the following questions:

Does an individual's personality type have an impact on their health status?
Are happy, positive, forward-thinking individuals less likely to suffer from ill health?
Or, are you more likely to be healthy if you are risk-averse and cautious?
What (if anything) does research tell us about the differences between optimists and pessimists
  with regard to health outcomes?

Modifiable Risk Factors

There is little we can do to alter our non-modifiable risk factors, but behaviour or lifestyle factors are something that we can influence. These are termed modifiable risk factors. The same behavioural factors, for example, smoking, high fat diets leading to high cholesterol levels, obesity and lack of physical activity, cause much of the early death and disability worldwide. In addition, consequences of such behavioural factors can also lead to high blood pressure and diabetes, themselves risk factors for developing CVD, vascular dementia and Alzheimer's disease (Alzheimer's Society UK 2016). A large research study examining the prevalence of CVD across high-, middle- and low-income countries found that 70% of all cases and deaths could be attributed to modifiable risk factors, with the most significant factor being high blood pressure (Yusuf et al. 2020). High blood pressure or, to give it its medical term, hypertension is largely a result of modifiable risk factors such as eating a high fat and high salt diet, being overweight or obese, smoking, alcohol consumption and lack of physical activity (WHO 2021d). Cancer is also associated with obesity, smoking and excessive alcohol use (Cancerdata 2023). This commonality of causes for the main killers is the reason that so much work is devoted to combatting these particular risk factors, either by working directly with people on individual behaviour change or by addressing societal measures which influence these factors.

High Blood Pressure (Hypertension)

High blood pressure is often termed 'a silent killer' because although it is extremely serious, it has no symptoms. It is estimated that 46% of adults with hypertension are undiagnosed, mainly those living in poor or low-income countries (WHO 2021d). However, the British Heart Foundation estimates that 4 million UK citizens under the age of 65 years have undiagnosed and therefore untreated hypertension (BHF 2019). High blood pressure can damage artery walls and increase the risk of developing the blood clots which cause heart attacks and strokes. It is also a significant risk factor for kidney disease. Adults should have a blood pressure of no more than 140 mm Hg systolic over 90 mm Hg diastolic (NICE.org.uk 2019). High blood pressure can be well controlled and brought down to normal limits with anti-hypertensive medications which have proven effectiveness if taken correctly. It is important, therefore, for adults, especially those over 40 years of age, to get checked every few years. Those already diagnosed with high blood pressure need checks at least yearly to ensure the medication prescribed is working effectively to keep BP within normal levels (NICE.org.uk 2019).

Smoking

Smoking detrimentally affects every organ of the body and is a leading risk factor for cancer, high blood pressure, IHD, stroke, lung diseases including chronic obstructive pulmonary disease (COPD) and diabetes. It also contributes to an increased risk of tuberculosis and immune disorders such as rheumatoid arthritis (Centres for Disease Control Tobacco Free 2017). There is no safe level of tobacco use and on an average smokers will die at least ten years earlier than non-smokers, with those starting smoking before the age of 15 doubling their chance of premature death (Ox.ac.uk 2020). Despite year-on-year reduction in smoking prevalence, in 2019 in the UK 14% of the adult population (those over 18) were still smoking regularly, with those in the 25–34 age bracket smoking the most at 19% (Windsor-Shellard 2020). Those working in manual and low-income employment were two and a half times more likely to smoke than those in professional occupations, and more than half of all current smokers expressed the desire to quit (Windsor-Shellard 2020). Globally, however, the picture is much worse with rates of tobacco use increasing in low- and middle-income countries. These countries account for 80% of all tobacco users worldwide (WHO 2021c). Recent years have seen a growth in e-cigarette use, with manufacturers citing their use in aiding smoking cessation and pointing to the fact that they are cleaner than cigarettes which contain high levels of additional toxins. E-cigarettes contain nicotine, the addictive part of cigarettes, so it seems logical to suggest that these are also addictive (McNeill et al. 2018). Nevertheless, the National Health Service (NHS) in England is considering providing medically licensed e-cigarettes as part of its smoking cessation arsenal (GOV.UK 2021). In 2019, it was estimated that there were 3,000 e-cigarette vaping stores in Britain, with e-cigarettes appearing to have a role more as a lifestyle product rather than a smoking cessation aid (Ashton 2019). Worryingly, e-cigarette use appears to be a fashionable trend in young people; 2% of 12-year-olds are said to use them, with the rates increasing with age, rising to 13% of 15-year-old boys and 9% of 15-year-old girls in England in 2018 stating that they were regular users (CMO 2020). It may be possible that e-cigarettes could become an entry level to smoking actual cigarettes, although research has shown that only 1% of children who vape have not previously smoked, so the two seemed linked (Public Health England 2020). The good news is that like the adult population smoking rates in young people continue to decline (CMO 2020).

High Blood Cholesterol

Having a high level of circulating blood cholesterol causes fatty deposits to be lain down in arteries, narrowing them and therefore making them susceptible to being blocked by blood clots, causing a heart attack or stroke. Levels of blood cholesterol are partly caused by a diet high in saturated fat (for example, from meat and dairy products) and also levels of cholesterol produced by the body itself in the liver (Lecerf and de Lorgeril 2011; NICE.org.uk 2021; Stone and Lloyd-Jones 2015). Some people produce excessive amounts of blood cholesterol, regardless of their diet and there is a genetic link to this, so it is common in some families (Bhatnagar, Handrean and Durrington 2008). Having a diet low in saturated fat and increasing exercise have been shown to reduce cholesterol levels. It is also important for adults to have regular cholesterol checks. UK guidelines state that adults should have a total cholesterol level of 5mmol/litre or below, with a low density lipoprotein (LDL) level of no more than 2 mmol/litre. LDL, sometimes referred to as the 'bad' cholesterol, is the cholesterol which creates fatty plaques in the arteries. Studies show that for every 1 mmol/litre reduction in LDL, there is a consequent 21% reduction in the risk of having a heart attack or stroke (NICE.org.uk 2021; Stone and Lloyd-Jones 2015;). Statin medication, which reduces cholesterol levels, has proved a very well tolerated and effective way of reducing the risk of CVD, as well as reducing the risk of another heart attack in those already affected (NICE.org.uk 2021). The good news is that partly as a result of the wider use of statins in recent years, levels of blood cholesterol have been falling in UK adults with the largest reduction being in those over 65 years and consequently at greatest risk of cardiovascular events (CMO 2020).

Diabetes

People who have diabetes are two to four times more likely to develop CVD and also to suffer from these conditions at an earlier age than the rest of the population (Leon 2015; National Institute of Diabetes and Digestive and Kidney Diseases [NIDDK] 2022). People with type 2 diabetes also tend to have other risk factors for developing CVD such as obesity, high cholesterol and lack of regular exercise. Hypertension is more than twice as common in people with diabetes as in people with normal blood glucose levels. Uncontrolled regulation of blood sugar causes damage to blood vessels, making them more prone to damage from atherosclerosis and hypertension (World Heart Federation 2013).

Poor Diet

A diet high in saturated fat leads to high circulating cholesterol levels in the blood and increases the laying down of fatty plaques in the arteries. A diet poor in fruit and vegetables leads to increased calorie intake from other sources and therefore risk of obesity. Fruit and vegetables have also been shown to have a protective effect against both CVD and cancer and people are encouraged to eat at least five portions per day (BHF 2022a; Casas et al. 2018). Diets high in salt (above four grams a day) found in quantities in processed food increase the risk of developing high blood pressure (NICE.org.uk 2021). Diets high in fibre have been proved to reduce cholesterol levels and eating oily fish twice a week has also been shown to reduce rates of CVD (Ignarro 2007). Other possible components of the diet such as soya products and nuts have been shown to be beneficial as the inclusion of these in the diet means less calories are obtained from saturated fat. It also follows that diets high in sugar due to the high concentration of calories in easily consumed small amounts of food can contribute to an increased risk of obesity as well as tooth decay.

Obesity

Being overweight affects the health of individuals in a myriad of ways. First, it puts them at the risk of hypertension, diabetes and atherosclerosis, which, in turn, can lead to CVD. Obese individuals can also suffer from sleep apnoea and musculoskeletal problems due to excess wear and tear on joints. It causes erectile dysfunction in men and stress incontinence in women and many gastrointestinal problems. There is also the issue of psychological and social difficulties caused by altered body image and stigma (NICE.org.uk 2014). A simple, although not entirely foolproof, method of measuring obesity is the calculation of a person's body mass index, the formula for this being kg/m^2, that is, dividing the person's weight in kilograms by the square of their height in meters. The subsequent score places the person in a weight category: underweight = <18.5, normal weight = 18.5–24.9, over-weight = 25–29.9, obese = BMI of 30 or greater (NICE.org.uk 2014). The UK has the second highest obesity rate in the world, following the USA. In 2020, more than 64% of the UK adult population was considered to be either overweight or obese. Of these, one in eight or 3.3% were considered to be morbidly obese with BMIs of over 40, which has been shown to reduce lifespan by 8–10 years (NHS Digital 2021). Childhood obesity is also rising. In 2020, 35% of children aged 10–11 years were found to be either overweight or obese (NHS Digital 2021). Research has uncovered ethnic differences regarding the risk of obesity and those of South Asian heritage run greater risks of developing CVD and diabetes. The BMI parameter of obesity for this population group has been set lower at 25 or above (BHF 2022b; World Heart Federation 2013). Central obesity (waist size) has been shown to influence the risk of developing CHD. High levels of abdominal fat can increase the production of dangerous LDL cholesterol. For this reason, it is recommended that men do not have a waist size of more than 40 inches (102 cm), and women's waist size should be 35 inches (88 cm) or less. For South Asian men and women, again, the recommended measurements are reduced to 36 inches (90 cm) and 32 inches (80 cm), respectively (BHF 2022b). A range of measures are in place to tackle obesity, for example, clearer food labelling, bans on certain food advertisements especially to children, industry standards and commitments to reduce sugar and salt in food and reduce buy one get one free promotions, increase access to weight management programmes and better training for health and care professionals, to mention just a few (Obesity Health Alliance 2021).

Lack of Exercise

The WHO states that physical inactivity has now become the fourth leading cause of global mortality. It contributes to a rising burden of disease, especially breast and colon cancer, diabetes and CHD (WHO 2020). The Chief Medical Officer's Annual Report in 2020 showed that in the UK, two thirds of adults were physically active, but that activity levels were significantly lower in more deprived populations, in older people and amongst the disabled or those with a chronic health condition (CMO 2020). The UK guidelines on physical activity are taken from the WHO report and state that adults between 19 and 64 years should do 150 minutes or two and a half hours of moderate intensity activity throughout the week in bursts of 10 minutes or more. Moderate activity is described as that which makes the individual slightly out of breath, brisk walking, cycling or swimming for instance. Alternatively, they may choose to do 75 minutes of more vigorous activity such as jogging or team sports (Department of Health [DH] 2011). In addition, adults should undertake muscle building exercise such as carrying shopping or working with weights at least two days a week and generally reduce sedentary behaviour. Children from 5 to 18 years are recommended to undertake at least an hour of moderate to vigorous activity every day and also to undertake muscle strengthening exercise or sports (DH 2011). Physical activity is beneficial as it maintains energy balance and helps prevent obesity. It also reduces the risk of coronary heart disease and stroke, diabetes, hypertension, colon cancer, breast cancer and depression. Additionally, it has been shown to have both preventative and therapeutic effects on musculoskeletal disorders such as osteoarthritis, osteoporosis and low back pain (WHO 2020). There are also more studies suggesting that physical activity is a protective factor for Alzheimer's disease and dementia by reducing cognitive decline in older adults (Buchman 2019; Horowitz 2020).

Alcohol Consumption

In the UK, the recommended maximum units of alcohol to lessen the chance of serious disease is 14 units per week for both men and women (NHS 2022). It is also recommended that people have one or two alcohol free days each week. It needs to be pointed out though that alcohol is closely associated with 60 different conditions and there is no completely safe level of consumption (WHO 2018). Half of the world's population does not drink at all and Western nations especially have a high level of alcohol-related harm (WHO 2018). Rather than the stereotypical perception that excess drinking occurs in young people, the facts show the excessive alcohol consumption in England is more likely to occur in middle-aged adults, with affluent men aged 55–65 drinking the most. Conversely, alcohol use in young people has been falling (CMO 2020). Regularly exceeding maximum recommended levels of consumption puts individuals at increased risk of alcoholic liver disease (accounting for 77% of all deaths in the UK related to alcohol), high blood pressure leading to heart attacks and strokes, mouth and throat cancer, and in women breast cancer. In addition, those drinking over the recommended levels are more likely to suffer from depression, weight gain (alcohol being high in calories), poor sleep and sexual problems (House of Commons Library 2021).

Drug Misuse

Since 2014, deaths from drug misuse have been increasing sharply in England, although there is much regional variation (CMO 2020). In 2019, a worldwide drug report published by the United Nations showed that 35 million people across the world suffered from drug misuse, but only one in seven was receiving treatment. Although cannabis remains the most widely used drug worldwide, opioid drug use is increasing and was responsible for two thirds of drug-related deaths in 2017. Cocaine production is rising steeply, but there is also a significant problem with synthetic opioids, especially in the USA (United Nations Office on Drugs and Crime 2019).

Stress

Whether long term or chronic stress increases the risk of CVD has been debated for some time, but more research is showing the link between high stress levels and various diseases. It has been suggested that stress may worsen inflammation in coronary arteries, leading to blood clots. Also, the release of the hormone cortisol which occurs in stressful situations has been linked with increasing the laying down of fat in the body (Sher 2005; Song et al. 2019; Tawakol et al. 2017). Being less able to cope with everyday pressures or distressing life events makes individuals less likely to adopt healthy behaviours and more likely to smoke more, drink more alcohol and eat more food, all of which can lead to an increased risk of CVD. In addition, stress is also being cited as a risk factor for Alzheimer's disease (Bisht, Sharma and Tremblay 2018; Machado et al. 2014), gastrointestinal disorders, eczema and psoriasis, inflammatory bowel disease, asthma and metabolic disorders (Liu, Wang and Jiang 2017; Sgambato et al. 2017). The mechanism is yet to be fully understood, but appears to be linked with the body's inflammatory response which is triggered by stress. In order to lessen stress, individuals need to be aware of the factors which cause them stress (known as stressors) and take measures to remove or lessen these if possible. Individuals should examine their workload, whether at work or in their home life, and be aware of taking too much on and striving too hard. Fostering mutually supportive relationships, undertaking enjoyable activities and taking time to relax and socialise are essential stress relievers. There are many relaxation techniques individuals may like to try, listening to soothing music or meditating to give themselves a period of relaxation each day (Varvogli and Darvirir 2011). Regular exercise and being outdoors can also help as a stress reliever and help to aid sleeping (Ewert and Chang 2018).

Activity

Using the link below, access session 4, pages 24–26 of the British Heart Foundation online training programme entitled Modifiable and Non-Modifiable Risk Factors. Follow the instructions to complete this short package, you may wish to do this individually or as an exercise to practice your group teaching skills.
https://www.bhf.org.uk/~/media/files/publications/healthy-hearts-and-chest-pain-kits/4-6-risk-factors-for-chd.pdf

---

Key Messages

- Although generally life expectancy is increasing worldwide, the gap between life expectancy and healthy life expectancy remains.
- Cardiovascular disease, chronic pulmonary disease and cancer are common causes of death worldwide.
- Developed nations are seeing an increased incidence of Alzheimer's disease and vascular dementia, whereas developing nations still suffer from diseases related to poverty such as diarrhoeal disease, tuberculosis and high maternal and infant mortality.
- Much chronic disease can be lessened by tackling modifiable risk factors.

References

All Party Parliamentary Group for Longevity. (2021). All Party Parliamentary Group for Longevity [online]. Available at: https://appg-longevity.org/levelling-up-health.

Alzheimer's Society UK. (2016). *Risk factors for dementia* [online]. Available at: https://www.alzheimers.org.uk/sites/default/files/pdf/factsheet_risk_factors_for_dementia.pdf

Alzheimer's Society. UK (2020). *Worst hit: Dementia during coronavirus* [online]. Available at: https://www.alzheimers.org.uk/sites/default/files/2020-09/Worst-hit-Dementia-during-coronavirus-report.pdf.

American Heart Association. (2021). *Understand your risks to prevent a heart attack* [online]. Available at: https://www.heart.org/en/health-topics/heart-attack/understand-your-risks-to-prevent-a-heart-attack

Ashton, J. (2019). Framing the question: Electronic cigarettes and harm reduction. *Journal of the Royal Society of Medicine*, 112(11), pp. 485–486.

Bhatnagar, D., Handrean, S. and Durrington, P. (2008). Hypercholesterolaemia and its management. *British Medical Journal*, 337, p. a993.

Bisht, K., Sharma, K. and Tremblay, M. (2018). Chronic stress as a risk factor for Alzheimer's disease: Roles of microglia-mediated synaptic remodeling, inflammation, and oxidative stress, *Neurobiology of Stress*, 9, 9–21. doi: 10.1016/j.ynstr.2018.05.003.

British Heart Foundation (BHF). (2019). *Four million people are living with untreated high blood pressure, new estimates show* [online]. Bhf.org.uk. Available at: https://www.bhf.org.uk/what-we-do/news-from-the-bhf/news-archive/2019/may/four-million-people-are-living-with-untreated-high-blood-pressure

British Heart Foundation (BHF). (2021). *Risk factors* [online]. Available at: https://www.bhf.org.uk/informationsupport/risk-factors

British Heart Foundation (BHF). (2022a). *Healthy eating*. Available at: https://www.bhf.org.uk/informationsupport/support/healthy-living/healthy-eating

British Heart Foundation (BHF). (2022b). *South Asian background and heart health*. Available at: https://www.bhf.org.uk/informationsupport/heart-matters-magazine/medical/south-asian-background

Buchman, A.S. (2019). Physical activity, common brain pathologies, and cognition in community-dwelling older adults. *Neurology*, 92, pp. 1–12. doi: 10.1212/WNL.0000000000006954.

Cancerdata. (2023). *English cancer prevalence statistics 2019*. Available at: https://www.cancerdata.nhs.uk/prevalence

Casas, R., Castro-Barquero, S., Estruch, R. and Sacanella, E. (2018). Nutrition and cardiovascular health. *International Journal of Molecular Sciences*, 19(12), 3988. doi: 10.3390/ijms19123988.

Centers for Disease Control and Prevention. (2021). *Injuries and violence are leading causes of death*. Available at: https://www.cdc.gov/injury/wisqars/animated-leading-causes.html

Centres for Disease Control Tobacco Free. (2017). *Health effects* [online]. Centers for Disease Control and Prevention. Available at: https://www.cdc.gov/tobacco/basic_information/health_effects/index.htm

Chief Medical Officer's (CMO) Annual Report. (2020). *Health trends and variation in England* [online]. GOV.UK. Available at: https://www.gov.uk/government/publications/chief-medical-officers-annual-report-2020-health-trends-and-variation-in-england.

Department of Health (DH). (2011). Physical activity guidelines for adults (19–64 years). Available at: http://www.dh.gov.uk/prod_consum_dh/groups/dh_digitalassets/documents/digitalasset/dh_128145.pdf

Diabetes UK. (2021). *Diabetes risk factors*. [online]. Available at: https://www.diabetes.org.uk/preventing-type-2-diabetes/diabetes-risk-factors

Ewert, A. and Chang, Y. (2018). Levels of nature and stress response. *Behavioral Sciences*, 8(5), p. 49. doi: 10.3390/bs8050049.

GOV.UK. (2021). *E-cigarettes could be prescribed on the NHS in world first*. Available at: https://www.gov.uk/government/news/e-cigarettes-could-be-prescribed-on-the-NHS-in-world-first.

Horowitz, A.M. (2020). Blood factors transfer beneficial effects of exercise on neurogenesis and cognition to the aged brain. *Science*, 369(6500), pp. 167–173. doi: 10.1126/science.aaw2622.

House of Commons Library. (2021). *Statistics on alcohol: England* [online]. Available at: https://researchbriefings.files.parliament.uk/documents/CBP-7626/CBP-7626.pdf

Ignarro, L. (2007). Nutrition, physical activity, and cardiovascular disease: An update. *Cardiovascular Research*, 73(2), pp. 326–340.

King's Fund. (2021). *What is happening to life expectancy in England?* [online]. Available at: https://www.kingsfund.org.uk/publications/whats-happening-life-expectancy-england#:~:text=By%202019%2C%20life%20expectancy%20at,level%20of%20a%20decade%20ago.

Lecerf, J.M. and de Lorgeril, M. (2011). Dietary cholesterol: From physiology to cardiovascular risk. *British Journal of Nutrition*, 106(1), pp. 6–14.

Leon, B.M. (2015). Diabetes and cardiovascular disease: Epidemiology, biological mechanisms, treatment recommendations and future research. *World Journal of Diabetes* [online], 6(13), p. 1246. Available at: https://www.ncbi.nlm.nih.gov/pmc/articles/PMC4600176/

Limb, M. (2021). Covid-19: Pandemic reduced life expectancy in most developed countries, study finds. *BMJ* [online], p. n2750. Available at: https://www.bmj.com/content/375/bmj.n2750

Liu, Y., Wang, Y. and Jiang, C. (2017). Inflammation: The common pathway of stress-related diseases. *Frontiers in Human Neuroscience*, 11. doi: 10.3389/fnhum.2017.00316.

Machado, A., Herrera, A.J., de Pablos, R.M., Espinosa-Oliva, A.M., Sarmiento, M., Ayala, A., Venero, J.L., Santiago, M., Villarán, R.F., Delgado-Cortés, M.J., Argüelles, S. and Cano, J. (2014). Chronic stress as a risk factor for Alzheimer's disease. *Reviews in the Neurosciences* [online], 25(6). Available at: https://www.degruyter.com/document/doi/10.1515/revneuro-2014-0035/html

McNeill, A., Brose, L.S., Calder, R., Bauld, L. and Robson, D. (2018). Evidence review of e-cigarettes and heated tobacco products 2018. Executive summary. Available at: https://www.issuesonline.co.uk/articles/evidence-review-of-ecigarettes-and-heated-tobacco-products-2018-executive-summary

National Institute of Diabetes and Digestive and Kidney Diseases (NIDDK). (2022). *Diabetes and health*. Available at: https://www.niddk.nih.gov/health-information/diabetes/overview/preventing-problems/heart-disease-stroke

NHS. (2022). *Alcohol units*. Available at: https://www.nhs.uk/live-well/alcohol-support/calculating-alcohol-units/

NHS Digital. (2021). *Statistics on obesity*. Available at: https://digital.nhs.uk/data-and-information/publications/statistical/statistics-on-obesity-physical-activity-and-diet/england-2020/appendices

NICE.org.uk. (2014). *Obesity: Identification, assessment and management guidance*. Available at: https://www.nice.org.uk/guidance/cg189/ifp/chapter/obesity-and-being-overweight

NICE.org.uk. (2019). *Recommendations | Hypertension in adults: Diagnosis and management | Guidance* [online]. NICE. Available at: https://www.nice.org.uk/guidance/ng136/chapter/recommendations

NICE.org.uk. (2021). *Lipid modification therapy for preventing cardiovascular disease*. Available at: https://pathways.nice.org.uk/pathways/cardiovascular-disease-prevention/lipid-modification-therapy-for-preventing-cardiovascular-disease.pdf

Obesity Health Alliance. (2021). *Turning the tide: A 10 year healthy weight strategy*. Available at: http://obesityhealthalliance.org.uk/turningthetide/

Office for National Statistics (ONS). (2020). *Life expectancy in the UK 2018-2020*. Newport: Office for National Statistics.

Office for National Statistics (ONS). (2021a). *Average age of those who had died with COVID-19*. Available at: https://www.ons.gov.uk/aboutus/transparencyandgovernance/freedomofinformationfoi/averageageofthosewhohaddiedwithcovid19

Office for National Statistics (ONS). (2021b). *Monthly mortality analysis, England and Wales*. Available at: https://www.ons.gov.uk/peoplepopulationandcommunity/birthsdeathsandmarriages/deaths/bulletins/monthlymortalityanalysisenglandandwales/august2021

Office for National Statistics (ONS). (2022). *Health and life expectancies*. Available at: https://www.ons.gov.uk/peoplepopulationandcommunity/healthandsocialcare/healthandlifeexpectancies

Ox.ac.uk. (2020). *Starting to smoke in childhood is much more dangerous than starting later* [online]. University of Oxford. Available at: https://www.ox.ac.uk/news/2020-05-21-starting-smoke-childhood-much-more-dangerous-starting-later

Public Health England. (2020). *Vaping in England: 2020 evidence update summary*. Gov.UK.

Qrisk.org. (2018). *QRISK3. Risk assessment tool for CHD* [online]. Available at: https://qrisk.org/three/index.php

Sgambato, D., Miranda, A., Ranaldo, R., Federico, A. and Romano, M. (2017). The role of stress in inflammatory bowel diseases. *Current Pharmaceutical Design* [online], 23(27). Available at: https://www.ingentaconnect.com/content/ben/cpd/2017/00000023/00000027/art00009

Song, H., Fang, F., Arnberg, F.K., Mataix-Cols, D., Fernández de la Cruz, L., Almqvist, C., Fall, K., Lichtenstein, P., Thorgeirsson, G. and Valdimarsdóttir, U.A. (2019). Stress related disorders and risk of cardiovascular disease: Population based, sibling controlled cohort study. *British Medical Journal*, 1255. doi: 10.1136/bmj.l1255.

Stone, N.J. and Lloyd-Jones, D.M. (2015). Lowering LDL cholesterol is good, but how and in whom? *New England Journal of Medicine*, 372(16), pp. 1564–1565.

Tawakol, A., Ishai, A., Takx, R.A., Figueroa, A.L., Ali, A., Kaiser, Y., Truong, Q.A., Solomon, C.J., Calcagno, C., Mani, V., Tang, C.Y., Mulder, W.J., Murrough, J.W., Hoffmann, U., Nahrendorf, M., Shin, L.M., Fayad, Z.A. and Pitman, R.K. (2017). Relation between resting amygdalar activity and cardiovascular events: A longitudinal and cohort study. *The Lancet*, 389(10071), pp. 834–845. doi: 10.1016/s0140-6736(16)31714-7.

United Nations Office on Drugs and Crime. (2019). *World Drug Report 2019: 35 million people worldwide suffer from drug use disorders while only 1 in 7 people receive treatment* [online]. Available at: https://www.unodc.org/unodc/en/frontpage/2019/June/world-drug-report-2019_-35-million-people-worldwide-suffer-from-drug-use-disorders-while-only-1-in-7-people-receive-treatment.html

Varvogli, L. and Darvirir, C. (2011). Stress management techniques: Evidence-based procedures that reduce stress and promote health. *Health Science Journal*, 5(2), pp. 74–89.

Windsor-Shellard, B. (2020). *Adult smoking habits in the UK* [online]. Available at: https://www.ons.gov.uk/peoplepopulationandcommunity/healthandsocialcare/healthandlifeexpectancies/bulletins/adultsmokinghabitsingreatbritain/2019#:~:text=In%20the%20UK%2C%20in%202019,2018%20to%2014.1%25%20in%202019 [accessed 29 October 2021].

World Bank. (2021). *Life expectancy at birth, total (years) | Data*. Available at: https://data.worldbank.org/indicator/SP.DYN.LE00.IN

World Health Organization (WHO). (2020). *Guidelines on physical activity and sedentary behaviour*. Available at: https://www.who.int/publications/i/item/9789240015128

World Health Organization (WHO). (2021a). *Global health estimates: Life expectancy and leading causes of death and disability*. Available at: https://www.who.int/data/gho/data/themes/mortality-and-global-health-estimates

World Health Organization (WHO). (2021b). *Suicide*. Available at: https://www.who.int/news-room/fact-sheets/detail/suicide

World Health Organization (WHO). (2021c). *Tobacco* [online]. Available at: https://www.who.int/news-room/fact-sheets/detail/tobacco

World Health Organization (WHO). (2021d). *Hypertension* [online]. Available at: https://www.who.int/news-room/fact-sheets/detail/hypertension

World Health Organization (WHO). (2022). *Alcohol* [online]. Who.int. Available at: https://www.who.int/news-room/fact-sheets/detail/alcohol

World Heart Federation. (2013). *Diabetes*. Available at: http://www.world-heart-federation.org/cardiovascular-health/cardiovascular-disease-risk-factors/diabetes/

Yusuf, S., Joseph, P., Rangarajan, S., Islam, S., Mente, A., Hystad, P., Brauer, M., Kutty, V.R., Gupta, R., Wielgosz, A., AlHabib, K.F., Dans, A., Lopez-Jaramillo, P., Avezum, A., Lanas, F., Oguz, A., Kruger, I.M., Diaz, R., Yusoff, K. and Mony, P. (2020). Modifiable risk factors, cardiovascular disease, and mortality in 155 722 individuals from 21 high-income, middle-income, and low-income countries (PURE): A prospective cohort study. *The Lancet* [online] 395(10226), pp. 795–808. Available at: https://pubmed.ncbi.nlm.nih.gov/31492503/

3   Health Inequalities

Susan R. Thompson

The World Health Organization's (WHO's) constitution states that: *The enjoyment of the highest attainable standard of health is one of the fundamental rights of every human being without distinction of race, religion, political belief, economic or social condition* (WHO 2021). This is the concept of health equity, that everyone should have the opportunity to achieve their full health potential. Nevertheless, throughout the world, there exist huge discrepancies in the standard of health individuals can expect. This depends on which country you live in, where in that country you live, your gender, age, sexual orientation, ethnicity, level of education attainment and fundamentally your level of income. The WHO has estimated that those living in higher income countries can expect to live 19 years longer than those living in poorer countries. One example is that a child born in Sierra Leone has a life expectancy of just 50 years, while a child born in Japan could be expected to reach 84 years (WHO 2019). Health inequality is not just about comparing countries; differences occur at very local levels. In Glasgow, Scotland, male life expectancy decreases by two years at every station on the train line linking the most affluent area of the city with the poorest district, and in all this amounts to a difference of 14 years (Public Health Scotland 2021). Certain demographic groups, for example, the learning disabled, are particularly affected by this disparity, with their life expectancy in England being around 30 years less than the non-learning disabled population (King's Fund 2021a). Worldwide, children from the poorest 20% of households are twice as likely to die before the age of five years than those from the richest 20% of households, with those living in sub-Saharan Africa 14 times more likely to die before the age of five than in the rest of the world (WHO 2018). This difference is referred to as the social gradient of health, whereby the higher up the social scale people are, the better people's health tends to be. It is not a direct comparison between the rich and the poor, but a gradient, that is, those in the middle of the gradient have better health than those below and those at the top have better health than those in the middle (Marmot 2004). In Chapter 1, we examined the wider or social determinants of health, and the way in which such factors as the level of income, level of education, housing standards, working conditions, food security, ethnic background, housing and the environment we live in can significantly affect our health status. Many of these determinants are unequally distributed in society and are further compounded by a lack of access to quality health care and more susceptibility to poor health behaviours (King's Fund 2020, 2021b, 2021c).

UK Health Inequalities

The UK uses Indices of Multiple Deprivation to compare different parts of the country. Certain factors or indices in an area are taken into account, and these are average income,

DOI: 10.4324/9781003411321-3

employment figures, educational levels, workforce skills and training, health and disability levels, amount of crime, barriers to housing and services and the living environment. Each local authority area is then awarded a score, and the lower the score, the more deprived the area. Middlesbrough, Liverpool, Knowsley, Kingston upon Hull and Manchester are the local authorities with the highest proportions of neighbourhoods amongst the most deprived in England. Middlesbrough and Blackpool rank as the most deprived districts regarding income deprivation amongst children (Public Health England [PHE] 2021). From 2018 to 2019, 42.3% of all children and 67.7% of children in lone-parent households in England were living below the minimum income standard for healthy living, compared with 29.1% of working age adults and 18.2% of pensioners (PHE 2021). The gap between those living in more affluent areas and those in more deprived areas is increasing. In England, those living in the more affluent south of the country can expect to live ten years more for men and eight years more for women than those living in the poorer north. Rates of long-term illness and the percentage of lifespan spent in ill health are also affected by this north-south divide. In 2021, a UK government report showed that due to ill health amongst the workforce, there was a £13 million productivity gap or 30% less production in the north of the country compared to the south (All Party Parliamentary Group 2021). Generally, those living in England have better health than those living in Wales and Northern Ireland, with Scotland lagging behind and having the highest all-causes mortality in the UK and lowest life expectancy at 77 years on average, 2.5 years behind that of England (Office of National Statistics [ONS] 2020). If we examine the health of Black and minority ethnic groups in Western society, they generally have a worse health status than their white counterparts within the same country. Examples from the UK show that Black women are four times more likely than white women to die from pregnancy and childbirth (Birthrights.org.uk 2021), two to four times more likely to be diabetic (Diabetes UK 2021) and twice as likely to die from COVID-19 as the white population (PHE 2021). However, it is essential to delve deeper into the differences within this population rather than just looking at them as a homogeneous group, which they are not. Bangladeshi men living in England can expect to have ten years less to live in good health than the white population and people with Black African and Black Caribbean heritage are subject to eight times the number of community mental health orders than whites are (King's Fund 2021b). Conversely, the Chinese population in the UK enjoys relatively good health, possibly because it is made up of a high percentage of younger people and students, but it also may be related to affluence. Income variables show that both Chinese and Indian ethnic groups earn considerably more than the white population who in turn earns more than Black African and Afro-Caribbean groups and those of Bangladeshi heritage earning the least (ONS 2018). These are just some examples of a range of evidence which show the health inequalities within various population groups.

COVID-19

The COVID-19 pandemic had a determinantal effect on health equity, as well as directly causing death and disability (in the form of long COVID); it also significantly affected health care systems causing enormous backlogs and increased waiting times for patients requiring treatment for non-emergency care. In addition, fear dissuaded people from coming forward to seek diagnosis and treatment, thereby potentially worsening their condition. Lockdowns and COVID regulations resulted in social isolation, an increase in domestic abuse and mental health conditions, financial insecurity and income reduction (Blundell et al 2020; Health Foundation 2021). Death rates from COVID-19 in deprived areas and in those with a high ethnic population were double that of more affluent areas (King's Fund 2021c). Vaccine hesitancy, described as a combination of complacency around not being susceptible to the virus, lack of confidence in the vaccine and lack of convenience regarding obtaining the vaccine all compounded this situation (Butler 2022). Misinformation and malicious disinformation circulated on social media and unfortunately the socially excluded and those lacking trust in society were more susceptible to the scaremongering and hence were less likely to come forward for vaccination and therefore at greater risk (Centers for Disease Control and Prevention [CDC] 2021).

Critical Thinking

Vaccine hesitancy: There are many vaccinations and immunisations available for a range of conditions, but it is not uncommon for people to refuse these. Take some time out to think about and research vaccine hesitancy.

What are the scare stories you have heard?
Where do they come from?
Who is benefiting from the vaccine rollout? Are there any losers?
What is being done to increase the level of trust for those in power held by different population groups?
Some countries make vaccination or immunisation for certain conditions a legal requirement. What are the pros and cons of this approach?

The existence of high quality health care and excellent medical technology is not a predictor of a nation's health. The USA spends more than any other country on health care, almost $11,000 per person, per year, yet its average life expectancy is three years behind Sweden's which spends half that amount. Black men in Harlem have a lower life expectancy than men in Bangladesh, and babies born in the USA are twice as likely to die before their first birthday compared to babies born in Japan (Office for Economic Cooperation and Development [OECD] 2021).

There is a significant difference in the rates of depression between groups in the highest income bracket and those in the lowest, suggesting a direct link with socio-economic status. Research has shown that increased financial strain, poor living conditions, having a chronic long-term condition and a lack of resources lead to an increase in depression. There is also evidence that people in the lower socio-economic groups are prescribed more medication for depression yet have less consultations and less planned but more crisis-related hospital treatment than those in higher socio-economic groups (Health Foundation 2020). The relationship with socio-economic status is compounded by the fact that often people who suffer from mental health problems have high unemployment rates and often experience stigma and prejudice towards them, which in turn affects income (Brouwers 2020).

The Income Gap

There is no doubt about it that reducing health inequalities is a complex area as it involves so many factors and influences on health. Some academics have argued however that it is the income gap between the rich and the poor in society that is the most significant factor in causing health inequality. They claim that the differences seen in life expectancy between the rich and the poor are directly related to the way that wealth is distributed in society (Benzeval et al., 2014; Joseph Rowntree Foundation [JRF] 2021; Wilkinson and Pickett 2006). They argue that life expectancy, infant mortality, teenage pregnancy, mental illness, crime, educational attainment and social mobility are directly correlated with the level of income equality. It is suggested that increased income disparity between people in society leads to a lack of trust and involvement in the community by those at the bottom of the income bracket (Putman 2000; Wilkinson and Pickett 2006). Being at the bottom of the income scale in a society which values success and status, it is claimed, leaves people with low self-esteem and feelings of resentment and inferiority and increased stress (Marmot 2004; Wilkinson and Pickett 2006, 2010, 2019).

Tackling Health Inequalities in the UK

The extent of the differences in the health of various sections of UK society first came to the public's consciousness with the publication of the Black Report (1980). This used health statistics from 1971 to examine the link between social class and health and asked the question: are people poor because they are ill? Or ill because they are poor? It found alarming discrepancies. For example, it found that the death rate for manual workers was twice that as for professionals and that male infants born into lower working-class families were three times as likely to die as male infants born to professional parents. Health can be seen as a political football and ideologies of political parties strongly affect health policy. Hence, the Black Report which advocated structural changes in society was met with some hostility by the incoming Conservative government of Margaret Thatcher (Asthana and Halliday 2006). Little was done in response to it to create a more equal society, but primary care services were overhauled and given a more defined role in providing preventative services, a key recommendation of the report. However, it was the individual who was seen as the major change agent. The responsibility lay, it was stated, with them, not society, and they needed to adopt healthier behaviour. When the Labour government came to power in 1997, typically the emphasis shifted from the individual to society. The new administration set targets to reduce health inequalities and commissioned an Independent Inquiry into Health Inequalities, another significant report to provide the prevailing picture, this was the Acheson Report (Acheson 1998). This report cited 39 recommendations to combat poverty, increase income, educational attainment and employment levels, and improve housing, the environment and transport. Rather than concentrating on health services, it acknowledged the part that wider determinants of health play in influencing health status and recommended improving the standard of living of the poorest in society, which it claimed would significantly reduce health inequalities (Acheson 1998). As a result of the Acheson report, the government of the day published a raft of policy documents including the White Paper Saving Lives – Our Healthier Nation (Department of Health [DH] 1999) which advocated partnership working across all agencies to tackle health and health inequalities. Targets were set that by 2010 the differences in both regional life expectancy and infant mortality between manual classes and the rest of the population should be reduced by 10%. The main proposals to bring about changes in life expectancy from birth were to tackle the causes of cancer and coronary heart disease, the biggest killers and which are noticeably higher in areas of deprivation. This led to dedicated quit smoking clinics being set up by all health authorities, doctors' surgeries undertaking to screen for behavioural factors related to coronary heart disease and cancer and ensuring better control of hypertension and diabetes. The goal of reducing infant mortality saw the setting up of Sure Start centres, health and social care centres for families of children aged 0–4 years living in deprived areas. It also saw actions to reduce teenage pregnancy with a wave of sexual health clinics and initiatives aimed at young people.

In 2002, the government published its Cross-Cutting Review which examined spending on the whole range of government programmes in education, welfare, criminal justice, environment, transport and local government in order to put actions into place to tackle health inequalities. This led to the setting up of neighbourhood renewal funds to aid regeneration in poorer communities (DH 2002).

However, when an update on health inequalities was published in 2009, although the health of the nation had improved generally with life expectancy having increased and infant mortality having fallen in the intervening years, 'the gap between the worst off and the average has not narrowed', and there were still 'persistent inequalities in income, educational achievement, literacy, unemployment, local areas, anti-social behaviour and crime' (DH 2009, p. 1).

In 2010, Michael Marmot published his updated report on health inequalities commissioned by the outgoing Labour Government. It was called 'Fair Society Healthy Lives'. It drew up six main policy objectives that were needed to be fulfilled in order to reduce inequalities in health (Marmot 2010). These were as follows:

1 Give every child the best start in life
2 Enable all children, young people and adults to maximise their capabilities and have control over their lives
3 Create fair employment and good work for all
4 Ensure a healthy standard of living for all
5 Create and develop healthy and sustainable places and communities
6 Strengthen the role and impact of ill-health prevention

The report again advocated the need to tackle the social gradient of health and protect the vulnerable.

> 'Taking action to reduce inequalities in health does not require a separate health agenda, but action across the whole of society'.
> (Marmot 2010, executive summary, p. 10)

The chronic long-term sick are generally either unable to work or have erratic work patterns punctuated by bouts of ill health. Marmot stated that the health gap should be narrowed through a mixture of increased taxation and increased welfare benefits or reducing pay differentials to become more in line with previous levels; a more equal society, he stated, would result in a healthier society. Economic benefits for the whole of society that would result if a reduction in health inequalities were accomplished resulting in increased productivity and tax revenue and lesser sickness benefit payments and treatment costs (Marmot 2010). The need for partnership working across local and national government agencies, the NHS and private and voluntary sectors was stressed in order to achieve widespread joined-up delivery of projects and initiatives.

In 2010, on the back of the worldwide financial crisis, the Conservative and Liberal Democrat UK government under David Cameron severely cut the financial benefits budget to the poorest in society, resulting in an estimated £14 billion reduction in the social welfare budget during the following ten-year period (New Economics Foundation 2021). Changes included a limit on maximum benefits per household and the number of dependent children able to be claimed for, a limit on housing allowances and the mean testing of child benefit payments (Roberts et al. 2014; Shildrick 2012). The criteria for disability benefits were also altered, targeting only those most in need, hence reducing benefits to disabled people by £5 billion (Disabilityrightsuk.org 2018). When changes are enacted in this way, the word 'reform' tends to be used by governments as it is associated with more positive connotations than 'cuts' and implies a change for the better. The WHO notes that it is only in times of greater liberality and affluence that there is a commitment to empowerment and equality (WHO 1999).

The widespread cuts in the benefit system in Western Europe and the USA following the financial crisis have resulted in detrimental health outcomes for the poorest in society (Health Equity.org. 2020; Shahidi et al. 2020).

A ten-year review of the Marmot report was published in 2020 which again stated that:

'The public and political debate on health needs to move towards the social determinants and away from the overwhelming focus on individual behaviours and health care'.

(Health Equity.org 2020, Executive Summary, p. 8)

The intervening period between both reports has seen an increase in food poverty with a proliferation of food banks and the rising cost of energy creating numerous press reports of people having to make the uncomfortable decision as to whether to heat their homes or to eat (Alderson 2022; Long 2022; Plummer 2022). Food poverty, a term unheard of in the UK in the late twentieth century, seems to be endemic in the twenty-first century (Enuf.org. uk 2017; The Trussell Trust 2021).

Levelling Up

In 2021, the UK Conservative Government launched its new Levelling Up agenda in another attempt to combat inequalities. It acknowledged the significant differences between regions in England and especially the difference between the affluent London and South-East which accounts for 40% of England's productivity and other parts of which have lower productivity levels than some Eastern European countries (Local.gov.uk 2021). It committed a total of £4.8 billion to increase the educational level and career opportunities to address economic disparity and for increased green space and leisure opportunities. A key tenet was to provide local government with more devolved taxation powers with a view to enable them to raise money and fund initiatives targeted at their specific communities (Local.gov. uk 2021). It remains to be seen whether this funding will readdress the substantial 77% cut to local government allocations from the national Ministry of Housing, Communities and Local Government between 2009–2010 and 2018–2019 (Health Equity.org 2020). However, it may be the case that the link between health status and income is finally being acknowledged and that as well as targeting health services the government is recognising that individual and community economic circumstances are as important. A recent NHS report 'Health as the New Wealth' (NHS Confederation 2020) specifically linked health status to economic status. The Joseph Roundtree Foundation is a long-standing think tank which has a high reputation for tackling social issues and inequalities. It publishes annual reports. Its 2021 report mirrored earlier recommendations to address inequalities in health. It specifically advised that the following are needed:

Good jobs paying a living wage.
Better employment opportunities for those with a disability and their carers.
A benefit system which supports people and is considered by society to be an essential tenet of a functional and caring society.
Affordable and secure housing.

(JRF 2021)

Although women tend to live longer than men, a greater proportion of their lifespan is spent in ill health. In 2022, the UK government published its first ever Women's Health Strategy for England to tackle the gender health gap. It is disconcerting that it took until 2022 to acknowledge and act on this (GOV.UK 2022). The strategy promises to increase access to breast cancer screening, fertility treatments and better understanding and training for doctors on women's health issues such as menopause with more research into women's health.

Activity

A comparison of the health status of the population of Blackburn with Darwen, a deprived area of North West England, with Windsor and Maidenhead, an affluent area of South-East England.

- Visit the Public Health Profiles Page at https://fingertips.phe.org.uk/
- Under National Public Profiles, select Local Authority Health Profiles
- Under Select a Region, select North-West, then Blackburn with Darwen and view data
- Click on the legend to show the key to the table
- Answer these questions:
- Is the life expectancy from birth of males getting better or worse? How does this compare to the national average for England shown as the red line down the centre of the diagram?
- Click on the topic tab and select other aspects of health such as behavioural factors, injuries and ill health, child health etc. to view these statistics. Are there any success stories?
- Go back to the Local Authority Health Profiles page and select South-East region, then select Windsor and Maidenhead.
- Compare the results you obtain from this area with the ones you obtained from Blackburn. Are there any surprises?
- What does this tell you about the link between health outcomes and deprivation?

Key Messages

- Worldwide inequalities in health persist both between countries and within countries.
- Social determinants of health such as level of income, level of education, housing standards, working conditions, food security, housing and the environment we live in can significantly affect our health status.
- In the UK, there is both a north-south divide and an income divide which means those in poorer areas of the country and those with less income have worsening health status than those in the south and those on higher incomes.
- There have been many reports and initiatives to reduce health inequalities, although these have had so far limited success, and health inequalities still persist in both developing and developed nations.

References

Acheson, D. (Chair). (1998). *Independent inquiry into inequalities of health*. London: The Stationery Office.

Alderson, L. (2022). *We have to decide between heating and eating because of rocketing energy bills...* [online]. The Sun. Available at: https://www.thesun.co.uk/money/17249019/decide-between-heating-eating-energy-bills/

All Party Parliamentary Group for Longevity. (2021). *All Party Parliamentary Group for Longevity* [online]. Available at: https://appg-longevity.org/levelling-up-health.

Asthana, S. and Halliday, J. (2006). *What works in tackling health inequalities: Pathways, policies and practice through the lifecourse*. Bristol. The Policy Press.

Benzeval, M., Bond, L., Campbell, M., Egan, M., Lorenc, T., Petticrew, M. and Popham, F. (2014). How does money influence health? Available at: https://www.jrf.org.uk/sites/default/files/jrf/migrated/files/income-health-poverty-full.pdf

Birthrights.org.uk. (2021). *New MBRRACE report shows Black women still four times more likely to die in pregnancy and childbirth - Birthrights* [online]. Birthrights. Available at: https://www.birthrights.org.uk/2021/11/11/new-mbrrace-report-shows-black-women-still-four-times-more-likely-to-die-in-pregnancy-and-childbirth/ [accessed 24 March 2023]

Black Report. (1980). *Inequalities in health, report of a research working group*. Chair Sir Douglas Black. London: DHSS.

Blundell, R., Costa Dias, M., Joyce, R. and Xu, X. (2020). COVID-19 and inequalities. *Fiscal Studies*, 41(2), pp. 291–319. doi: 10.1111/1475-5890.12232

Brouwers, E.P.M. (2020). Social stigma is an underestimated contributing factor to unemployment in people with mental illness or mental health issues: Position paper and future directions. *BMC Psychology* [online], 8(1). Available at: https://bmcpsychology.biomedcentral.com/articles/10.1186/s40359-020-00399-0

Butler, R. (2022). Vaccine Hesitancy: What it means and what we need to know in order to tackle it. Available at https://www.who.int/immunization/research/forums_and_initiatives/1_RButler_VH_Threat_Child_Health_gvirf16.pdf

Centers for Disease Control and Prevention (CDC). (2021). *How to address COVID-19 vaccine misinformation* [online]. Centers for Disease Control and Prevention. Available at: https://www.cdc.gov/vaccines/covid-19/health-departments/addressing-vaccine-misinformation.html

Department of Health (DH). (1999). *Saving lives – Our healthier nation*. London. The Stationary Office.

Department of Health (DH). (2002). *Tackling health inequalities - 2002 cross-cutting review*. London. The Stationary Office.

Department of Health (DH). (2009). *Tackling health inequalities:10 years on, a review of developments in tackling health inequalities in England over the last 10 years*. London: The Stationary Office.

Diabetes UK. (2021). *Diabetes risk factors* [online]. Available at: https://www.diabetes.org.uk/preventing-type-2-diabetes/diabetes-risk-factors

Disabilityrightsuk.org. (2018). *Disability benefit spending reduced by £5 billion over the last decade | Disability Rights UK* [online]. Available at: https://www.disabilityrightsuk.org/news/2018/september/disability-benefit-spending-reduced-%C2%A35-billion-over-last-decade

Enuf.org.uk. (2020). *ENUF | Evidence and network on UK household food insecurity* [online]. Available at: https://enuf.org.uk

GOV.UK. (2022). *Women's health strategy for England* [online] Available at: https://www.gov.uk/government/publications/womens-health-strategy-for-england/womens-health-strategy-for-england#:~:text=The%20strategy%20builds%20on%20Our,care%20system%20listens%20to%20women

Health Equity.org. (2020). Health Equity in England: The Marmot Review in England 10 years on [online]. Available at: https://www.health.org.uk/sites/default/files/2020-03/Health%20Equity%20in%20England_The%20Marmot%20Review%2010%20Years%20On_executive%20summary_web.pdf

Health Foundation. (2020). *Inequalities in health care for people with depression and/or anxiety | The Health Foundation* [online]. Available at: https://www.health.org.uk/publications/long-reads/inequalities-in-health-care-for-people-with-depression-and-anxiety

Health Foundation. (2021). *Emerging evidence of health Inequalities and Covid 19*. Available at: https://www.health.org.uk/news-and-comment/blogs/emerging-evidence-on-health-inequalities-and-covid-19-march-2021

Joseph Rowntree Foundation (JRF). (2021). *UK poverty 2020/21* [online]. Available at: https://www.jrf.org.uk/report/uk-poverty-2020-21

King's Fund. (2020). *What are health inequalities?* Available at: https://www.kingsfund.org.uk/publications/what-are-health-inequalities

King's Fund. (2021a). *What is happening to life expectancy in England?* [online]. Available at: https://www.kingsfund.org.uk/publications/whats-happening-life-expectancy-england#:~:text=By%202019%2C%20life%20expectancy%20at,level%20of%20a%20decade%20ago

King's Fund. (2021b). *The health of people from ethnic minority groups in England* [online]. The King's Fund. Available at: https://www.kingsfund.org.uk/publications/health-people-ethnic-minority-groups-england#:~:text=Cardiovascular%20disease%202%20(CVD)%20is,poor%20outcomes%20from%20Covid-19 [accessed 26 October 2021].

King's Fund. (2021c). *Health inequalities in a nutshell* [online] Available at: https://www.kingsfund.org.uk/projects/nhs-in-a-nutshell/health-inequalities

Local.gov.uk. (2021). *Levelling up* [online]. Available at: https://www.local.gov.uk/about/campaigns/levelling#:~:text=The%20Levelling%20Up%20White%20Paper,all%20parts%20of%20the%20country

Long, J. (2022). *Heat or eat: Many forced to ration food and heating amid surging energy prices* [online]. Channel 4 News. Available at: https://www.channel4.com/news/heat-or-eat-many-forced-to-ration-food-and-heating-amid-surging-energy-prices

Marmot, M. (2004). *The status syndrome: How social standing affects our health and longevity.* London. Bloomsbury.

Marmot, M. (2010). *Fair society, healthy lives, strategic review of health inequalities in England post 2010*. Institute of Health Inequity.

New Economics Foundation. (2021). *How our benefits system was hollowed out over 10 years* [online]. Available at: https://neweconomics.org/2021/02/social-security-2010-comparison

NHS Confederation. (2020). *Health as the new wealth* [online]. Available at: https://www.nhsconfed.org/publications/health-new-wealth

Office for Economic Cooperation and Development (OECD). (2021). *Health resources – Health spending – OECD data* [online]. Available at: https://data.oecd.org/healthres/health-spending.htm

Office of National Statistics (ONS). (2018). *Annual population survey*. Available at: https://www.ons.gov.uk/searchdata?q=annual%20population%20survey

Office of National Statistics (ONS). (2020). *Life expectancy in the UK 2018- 2020*. Newport: Office of National Statistics.

Plummer, R. (2022). *Surging food prices push inflation to 30-year high* [online]. BBC News. Available at: https://www.bbc.co.uk/news/business-60050699

Public Health England (PHE). (2021). *Health Profile for England: 2021* [online]. GOV.UK. Available at: https://www.gov.uk/government/publications/health-profile-for-england-2021 [accessed 24 March 2023].

Public Health Scotland. (2021). *Measuring health inequalities* [online]. Healthscotland.scot. Available at: http://www.healthscotland.scot/health-inequalities/measuring-health-inequalities

Putman, R. (2000). *Bowling alone: The collapse and revival of American community*. New York: Simon & Schuster.

Roberts, E., Price, L. and Crosby, L. (2014). *Just about surviving: A qualitative study on the cumulative impact of welfare reform in the London borough of Newham*. Wave 2 Report. London: Community Links.

Shahidi, F.V., Muntaner, C., Shankardass, K., Quiñonez, C. and Siddiqi, A. (2020). The effect of welfare reform on the health of the unemployed: Evidence from a natural experiment in Germany. *Journal of Epidemiology and Community Health* [online], 74(3), pp. 211–218. Available at: https://jech.bmj.com/content/74/3/211.abstract

Shildrick, T. (2012). Low pay, no pay churning: The hidden story of work and worklessness. *Poverty*, 142, pp. 6–9.

The Trussell Trust. (2021). *State of hunger - The Trussell Trust* [online]. Available at: https://www.trusselltrust.org/state-of-hunger/

Wilkinson, R.G. and Pickett, K.E. (2006). Income inequality and health: A review and explanation of the evidence. *Social Science & Medicine*, 62(7), pp. 1768–1784.

Wilkinson, R.G. and Pickett, K.E. (2010). *The spirit level: Why equality is better for everyone*. London: Penguin.

Wilkinson, R.G. and Pickett, K.E. (2019). *The inner level: How more equal societies reduce stress, restore sanity and improve Everyone's well-being*. London. Penguin.

World Health Organization (WHO). (1999). *Healthy public policy: WHO health 21 targets 1 and 2*. Copenhagen: WHO Regional Office for Europe.

World Health Organization (WHO). (2018). *Health inequities and their causes* [online]. Who.int. Available at: https://www.who.int/news-room/facts-in-pictures/detail/health-inequities-and-their-causes

World Health Organization (WHO). (2019). *Social determinants of health* [online]. Who.int. Available at: https://www.who.int/health-topics/social-determinants-of-health#tab=tab_1

World Health Organization (WHO). (2021). *Constitution of the World Health Organization* [online]. WHO.int. Available at: https://www.who.int/about/governance/constitution

4 Approaches and Models Used to Promote Health

Susan R. Thompson

So far the discussion has centred around the complex nature of what influences health and how these influences combine to produce inequalities in health. Now it is time to move forward to examining what can be done and is being done to reduce these inequalities and improve the health status of individuals and communities. Much of the work comes under the heading of health promotion, which is described as 'The process of enabling people to increase control over the determinants of health and thereby improve their health' (World Health Organization [WHO] 1986).

Primary, Secondary and Tertiary Health Promotion

Health promotion interventions have been traditionally described as primary, secondary or tertiary (Deloitte Centre for Health Solutions 2022). Primary prevention is aimed at the risk factors which cause ill health and seeks to prevent ill health from starting in the first place, so typically it targets risk factors. As we have seen influences on health are wide ranging, primary prevention covers an exceptionally wide field. A few examples would be the provision of cycle lanes to cut down on death and injury for cyclists and tobacco control measures to reduce access. Secondary prevention is about identifying issues in the early stages whilst there is still time for a cure or mitigation of serious illness. Health screening for aortic aneurysm, breast cancer and inherited diseases would come under secondary prevention initiatives. Also in this category are behavioural interventions to stop risk factors leading to disease, for example, weight management, smoking cessation interventions and the use of medication such as statins to lower cholesterol. All such interventions seek to stop or slow the advance of disease. Tertiary health promotion steps in when disease is already present with the aim of reducing the complications and ongoing progression of the disease (Deliotte 2022). Some examples of how diseases are managed include chemotherapy for cancer, rehabilitation following a heart attack or stroke, physiotherapy and anti-inflammatory medication for arthritis. You will see that tertiary health promotion is closely aligned with medical treatment, but it takes a range of forms with many practitioners being involved, such as nurses, midwives, occupational therapists, dieticians and doctors. It is obviously better to prevent or limit risk factors from causing disease. So much of the work of health promotion is at the primary and secondary prevention levels. Unfortunately, money for preventative care in the UK has been falling in recent years. In 2013, spending on health care services stood at £6.8 billion, and only 5% of this was spent on prevention. However, the situation had gotten worse by 2019; health care spending had risen to £8 billion but the proportion spent on preventative services had reduced to 4.5% of the total (Office for National Statistics [ONS] 2021). Most of the

DOI: 10.4324/9781003411321-4

money spent is on the secondary and tertiary elements of health promotion and public health, and spending per capita of the population fell by almost a quarter between 2015 and 2022 (Deliotte 2022). The COVID-19 pandemic significantly reduced access to preventative services such as smoking cessation clinics and weight management programmes, further compounding this issue (Deliotte 2022).

Researchers and academics who study health promotion have identified common themes and key aspects which make up the totality of health promotion and hence seek to clarify the complex interplay of interventions used in practice. This is with a view to providing those tasked with planning health promotion interventions with information and guidance regarding effective practice. This information is characteristically presented as models or frameworks, often illustrated pictorially to aid understanding. Although many models have been devised, there is much overlap between them, so only a few will be presented within this text.

Five Approaches Commonly Used in Health Promotion

Ewles and Simnett were some of the earliest researchers to study the new discipline of health promotion. In their seminal work (Ewles and Simnett 2003), they discerned that in essence there are five approaches or types of intervention which ideally *in combination* can be used to bring about improvements in health both at an individual and a population level. These approaches are discussed in the following section and are still considered relevant and are used today throughout health promotion practice.

The Medical Approach

This involves the use of medical or clinical techniques to prevent ill health and reduce morbidity and premature mortality. Such interventions include health screening and monitoring, blood pressure checking or cervical smear down the line. The individual tests. It also includes the significant vaccination programmes in place aiming to prevent or limit the severity of a wide range of infectious diseases from whooping cough to hepatitis and COVID-19. Medication is used to prevent and control existing conditions, to prevent them from worsening and causing more severe symptoms and more serious health issues. Controlling diabetes by using insulin to maintain a satisfactory blood sugar level lessens the risk of diabetic complications and heart disease. This approach can also include surgical interventions and procedures such as gastric band surgery which reduces the size of the stomach in order to combat obesity or angioplasty to widen narrowed coronary arteries to prevent a heart attack.

The medical approach lends itself to testing via clinical trials more easily than the other approaches which occur in a less controlled environment, so the effectiveness of medical interventions can often be measured more easily. This credibility means the medical approach attracts greater funding than other more low-key interventions and is supported by big businesses such as pharmaceutical companies and medical equipment manufacturers. It is generally a very expensive approach. New medication, clinical procedures, laboratory tests and the utilisation of highly trained health professionals and the health service infrastructure are all costly. In the UK, the National Institute of Health and Care Excellence (NICE) carefully weighs up each proposed new intervention to decide whether the costs associated with it are worth the life years to be gained (NICE 2022). There comes the problem of managing public demand. Health care is an extremely important political responsibility and governments around the world need to ensure that it is adequately funded. Well informed sections of the public are alert to new drugs and procedures and could be a vocal force if services are withdrawn, so it's essential that before interventions are introduced, they have proven cost-effectiveness, are available to all and can be sustained long term.

Immunisation and Screening

Immunisations are an extremely effective way of combating the spread of infectious disease throughout populations. However, in order to have a significant effect on the incidence of disease at a population level, a significant number of people need to be immunised. Low take up of vaccinations prevent this population effect and lead to epidemics. This has been seen in recent years with the outbreaks of measles in the UK following scares around the measles, mumps and rubella (MMR) vaccination (Sathyanarayana Rao and Andrade 2011). This has been further compounded by the COVID-19 pandemic which reduced the number of children accessing health services for vaccination, thereby increasing the risk of outbreaks of measles and other childhood diseases (Torjesen 2021; WHO 2021). COVID-19 vaccination uptake has generally been very successful, although vaccine hesitancy persists particularly amongst certain ethnic groups. Amongst vaccination rates, inequalities persist, with the populations of the wealthier nations of the world receiving the most immunisation and the poorer countries, noticeably African nations, receiving the least coverage (Johns Hopkins Coronavirus Resource Center 2022).

Screening is an aspect of the medical approach which has expanded in recent years benefiting from research into the causes and markers of disease. Screening is now possible for a range of conditions throughout the life cycle, from screening of babies for Down's syndrome and cystic fibrosis, through breast and cervical screening, bowel cancer screening and the risk of developing a serious aortic aneurysm. Screening procedures vary in their level of invasiveness, from heel pricks in babies to mammograms in older women, but in order to be cost-effective, and to encourage uptake, screening needs to be specific, sensitive and safe. Specificity means that it should identify only those with the disease, and it shouldn't wrongly identify that someone has the disease when they don't. Sensitivity means that the screening should identify all those with the disease. It shouldn't miss anyone out and it should be safe; that is, it shouldn't cause problems for the individual, either through unnecessary anxiety or physical issues caused by the screening process. The NHS in England has rejected a nationwide screening test for prostate cancer as the test is not specific enough, with two out of three men with raised levels following the test not actually being shown to have cancer after further tests are carried out. The test also proved to lack sensitivity in the fact that it misses men with prostate cancer (NHS Choices 2022). In 2012, research showed that although mammography for breast cancer saved the lives of 1,300 women, an estimated 4,000 women probably underwent unnecessary chemotherapy and radiotherapy treatment for cancers which were too slow growing to ever cause them harm (Marmot et al. 2013). A separate study involving the Canadian service showed a similar finding by Seely and Alhassan (2018) that breast screening reduced mortality by 40%, but false positives occur in 10% of women and perhaps more worrying false negatives (i.e. cancer present but not detected) in up to 20% of women tested. This may give women a false sense of reassurance which in turn may lead them to ignore changes they themselves identify. Screening remains an extremely useful public health tool and is improving all the time; however, it is important to provide the public with the facts to make sure that they are aware of the pros and cons of entering into screening.

Behavioural Change

This is the approach which is possibly the most familiar and recognisable when thinking about health promotion. The onus of this approach is on individuals to change their behaviour, the behaviour which is deemed as being 'unhealthy' and results in them being classed as being 'at risk' of disease or injury or worsening health. Behaviours such as drinking too much alcohol, having unprotected sex, driving recklessly and being inactive are just a few examples from a myriad of behaviours that have been shown to have a negative effect on health status. The world's health care systems invest much time and effort in persuading us all to adopt healthier behaviours. After all, individuals choosing to lessen their risk of serious disease makes good economic sense, potentially resulting in huge cost savings in health care costs further down the line. The individual benefits too, of course, after quitting smoking people find that they feel fitter and are able to do more before becoming short of breath, their cough disappears, they have improvements in taste and smell, their hair is shiner and their complexion fresher. This is in addition to the reduction in risk of cancer and heart disease which occurs after quitting (Action on Smoking and Health 2020). Supporting individuals through behaviour change forms a core element of the roles of various professional and semi-professional health workers such as practice nurses, health visitors, smoking cessation advisers, community nutrition assistants and sexual health workers, and also those who work outside the health service such as sports development officers, youth workers and cycling officers. All such are tasked with facilitating healthy choices, providing information and equipment, working with individuals or groups to set goals and action plans and maintaining ongoing contact in order to support people through change. The development of these skills will be discussed in more detail in later chapters.

Behaviour change is essential if modern society is to combat the burden of disabling long-term conditions such as diabetes, chronic respiratory problems, coronary heart disease and stroke. However, for this approach to work successfully, resources do need to be invested in supporting people through such changes. Money needs to be spent on training and paying for advisers, venues and equipment such as carbon monoxide monitors or free condoms. Despite the potential for cost savings, a systematic review conducted in 2017 showed that since the worldwide economic recession of 2008, funding for health behaviour initiatives in high-income countries had been substantially reduced. The review showed that behavioural interventions provided an excellent return on investment and that cuts to such services represented a false economy (Masters et al. 2017).

Critical Thinking

Take some time out to think about and research the following:

What is meant by a return on investment in this context?
Is it just money saved that is considered here?
What other values and benefits need to be taken into consideration?
Are interventions that don't save money for health services still worth doing?

All too often judgemental statements are made against people whose behaviour is considered unhealthy which results in victim blaming. As has been discussed, behaviour is influenced by many factors. There needs to be an understanding by all health promoters that the relationship between the individual and the social environment is complex. Helping people to change involves making a proper assessment of the individual's circumstances and finding a plan of action which meets the goals they have set themselves and which is achievable for them. Relapse is common and again the reasons for this need to be understood and worked around. As an approach, evaluation of the effectiveness of specific interventions and services can be hard to prove because of the multiple factors at play in any successful or unsuccessful attempt at change. For example, if someone starts smoking again, this may be a reflection on the quit smoking service or the fact that their partner continues to smoke.

Educational Approach

Health education is the imparting of information regarding the causes of ill health and conversely what can be done in order to benefit health. As such it is an essential first step for individuals and communities wishing to improve their health. After all, if people aren't aware, for example, that using a condom protects against sexually transmitted disease, why would they be expected to use one. Health education takes many forms, from leaflets and posters in doctors' surgeries, to articles in magazines, posts on social media and even storylines in soap operas. Health education has the capacity to reach a large number of people, in this age of mass communication, never before have people been so well informed about health and the causes of disease; however, ignorance and misunderstandings persist. The role of health education will be discussed in more detail in Chapter 6, but the main issue with the educational approach is that although it is an essential first step, it is not an end in itself. Too often inexperienced health promoters feel that all that is required is the presentation to the public of cause and effect and that this will automatically lead individuals to undertake change. That, for example, if someone is aware of healthy levels of alcohol consumption and made aware of the risks associated with excess consumption, logically they will drink within normal limits. This of course is far too simplistic. Unfortunately, behaviour is influenced by many more things than just knowledge, so it is essential to combine the educational approach with other approaches.

Client-Centred or Empowerment Approach

The aim of this approach is to provide support to enable people and communities to take control of their health and set their own agenda which relates to their own interests and values regarding health. Individuals and community representatives are seen as partners with health promoters who act as facilitators and provide information, support and possibly help with funding and resources so that health priorities can be identified and action plans created to achieve the goals set. What is important within this approach is that it is the community or individual who decides on what the health need is, not the professional. Health promoters are often at the mercy of departmental or governmental targets to concentrate on a specific health issue; however, imposing a health priority which does not match the perceived need of the client is self-defeating, and telling people what is needed rarely works.

Conversely, working with a client's high motivation towards tackling a specific health issue will undoubtedly be more successful than imposing on them a health need which the client doesn't recognise or prioritise. Empowerment is more of an ethos or a key principle perhaps than an approach, a principle of enabling a power shift from the professional to the client which should underpin all interactions no matter what the health promotion intervention is (Kayser et al. 2019). Empowering people enables them to gain the knowledge and skills and assertiveness they require to make positive changes happen. Empowerment can be a long-term process so there are few quick wins and evaluation of effectiveness again can be difficult to prove. Empowerment is very much about the individual or community choosing their own agenda, which means that a variety of issues may be identified often at odds with the national or local agenda (WHO n.d.). A community group may feel, for example, that their priority is rejuvenating a piece of waste ground, possibly to make it into a play area, whereas the local health authority's public health agenda may be to combat the area's high rate of teenage pregnancy, an issue which may be of little concern to the residents. Widening the agenda can be seen as having a diluting effect and is the opposite of a concerted multifaceted campaign pinpointed towards one particular health issue which may result in a population-wide effect. Ways to promote empowerment will be discussed in more detail in later chapters.

Societal Change

This approach moves away from the individual to concentrate on society as a whole. The aim of the societal change approach is to bring about changes in the physical, social and economic environment in order to make healthy choices easier for people to make. The focus is on changing society and developing policies, guidelines and laws which promote health at local and national levels. As such individuals are not singled out and changes are made which tend to affect everyone; the law banning smoking in public places or rules about the wearing of face masks are such examples. Other examples include food labelling guidelines, housing standards and fluoridisation of the water supply. People can rarely opt out of these initiatives, they catch everyone and can directly or indirectly influence behaviour. It is the societal change approach that perhaps best tackles the wider determinants of health that were discussed in Chapter 1. As the societal change approach does not pinpoint individuals, it avoids victim blaming and as it captures everyone, it can result in widespread and effective change. A systematic review of 21 countries which had imposed a smoking ban in indoor places found that rates of coronary heart disease and stroke had reduced as had the severity of pulmonary diseases (National Institute for Health Research Evidence 2020). Such national changes obviously reach the whole population, but governments need to be careful; accusations of the state interfering too much with personal choices are often made. It is important that the public supports proposed public health measures, as if not the result could be severely disadvantageous to the political party imposing them. Consultations, adequate warning and information about proposed changes and what they mean and extra support put in place to ease people through change are all essential if the public is to concede and conform.

Although the approaches above are described separately, in practice the approaches are not mutually exclusive. Greater effectiveness results from all these approaches being used in combination with each other.

Activity

Considering the five approaches, think of interventions for each approach which are already used or could possibly be used to tackle the risk factors of coronary heart disease referred to in Chapter 2.

Examples are given in Table 4.1.

Top-Down or Bottom-Up

When studying the approaches referred to above, it can be seen that some approaches are more top-down, that is, in the control of the health professional or the state, the medical approach and the societal approaches, for example, whereas other approaches are more bottom-up (see Figure 4.1), that is, in the control of the client, the empowerment and behavioural change approaches being the obvious examples. There has been much debate regarding moving from a paternalistic system whereby clients largely have decisions about their health imposed on them to a system where people are encouraged to make their own choices about their health (Baum and Fisher 2014; Whitehead and Irvine 2010). In effect, these two opposites coexist within public health. Laws are passed which require total conformity. At the same time, competent health promoters work to help clients pursue action plans that they have identified, which may work for them. A key driver for governments around the world faced with the burden of increasing demands on health care systems is cost. Limiting the demand on health care systems by bringing about changes in individual behaviour that contribute to ill health is more cost-effective than spending money on health care (Deloitte Centre for Health Solutions 2022). Most health care systems are in part, if not totally, funded by taxation and there is always the political push to limit the tax burden on the population (Baggott 2010). The public are unwilling to pay the price of their neighbour's irresponsible lifestyle, and as knowledge has grown about the causes of disease, so has blame. Perhaps when someone died of a heart attack in 1870, the community might have been more

Table 4.1 Five Approaches Used to Tackle Coronary Heart Disease

Approach	Intervention
Medical	Use of medication to lower cholesterol and blood pressure. Screening for angina. Coronary artery bypass and angioplasty operations
Behavioural	Weight management and stop smoking clinics. Walking groups
Educational	Posters and websites providing information and tips on adopting a healthy lifestyle and signposting people to services. Television advertisements warning of the dangers of second-hand smoke. Articles in magazines and newspapers. Social media stories
Empowerment	Health promoters working with clients to identify and meet their specific health needs, for example, tackling weight loss before smoking if that is the client's priority
Societal change	Manufacturer agreements limiting the level of salt, sugar and fat in processed food. Investment in footpaths and cycle to work schemes. Policies on school playing fields and school meals

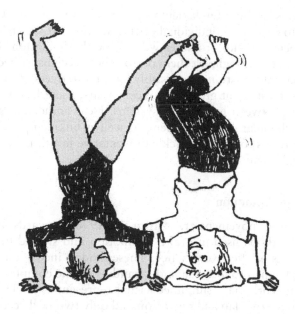

Are you sure that this is what they meant by 'be more bottom up?'

Figure 4.1 The Bottom-up Approach

sympathetic than today, when voices may be heard condemning the individual's obesity, smoking habit and lack of exercise. What is more, people who die early are taken out of the workforce. Those with a chronic illness may not be working and therefore not contributing to the economy either. Rather, they may be claiming disability benefits. All the above have resulted in governments taking charge and targeting ill health systematically through legislation, industry-wide agreements, health and safety policies, health screening, road traffic controls and a commitment to providing information to the public through websites and advertisement campaigns (Public Health England [PHE] 2019). There remains, however, the need for health promoters to adopt a bottom-up approach where the focus of intervention is directed by the client rather than the professional. In this the health promoter is often placed in a dilemma, as they are often a government employee; they are largely directed by priorities set by that government. Services are developed with priorities in mind. In the UK in the first decade of the 21st century, a tremendous push was instigated to reduce the number of smokers in the population in order to reduce levels of cancer and coronary heart disease. The Department of Health made £138m available over the three years from 2003 to 2006 to set up smoking cessation services nationwide, workers were trained, premises found, clinics set up and incentives adopted, such as free nicotine replacement therapy (Department of Health 2008). It can be inferred that as funding is directed to key target areas, this leaves less money for the priority of individual clients, should those not conform to the target areas. Despite exhortations to staff to work with the priorities of their clients, health promoters are constrained by funding and the limitation of their role. Smoking cessation advisers will have been employed to run a quit smoking clinic with expectations of a certain throughput of clients and success rate. They will have limited training or time to spend with individuals whose stress level is a fundamental reason why they are unable to quit smoking and no power at all to change the individual circumstances that the client finds themselves in. However, a competent health promoter will realise the limitations of the role and be able to fully assess clients and signpost them on to other specialist services should they exist. Voluntary and charitable institutions possibly have more freedom to concentrate on the priorities of their specialist client groups. In recent years, there has been a push towards collaborative working between health care systems, local authorities and the voluntary, charitable sectors. Such integrated care systems as well as linking up health and social care services also bring partners together to tackle preventative health issues and reduce health inequalities (The King's Fund 2021).

Models Used in Health Promotion

As the health promotion movement grew from the 1970s onwards, academics took an interest in studying methods used in health promotion and started to draw conclusions and recommend models of effective practice. These models incorporated the approaches mentioned above and aimed to increase understanding of the complex interplay of methods and ideologies at work via a simplified visual representation. There are many such models but there is much overlap and repetition and only two well-recognised models will be discussed here.

Beattie's Model of Health Promotion

Beattie's model acknowledged that approaches are either top-down or bottom-up, and these he calls authoritative (expert led) or negotiated (valuing the individual's autonomy) (Beattie 1991). The approaches he suggests are also aimed at individuals or communities. The left-hand side of the model deals with those interventions directed at individuals, whereas the right-hand side looks at more collective interventions. A continuum is used to express these concepts. The continuum is useful as in practice approaches blur and overlap as does often the focus of the intervention. Beattie doesn't use the Ewles and Simnett's approaches but identifies four different, yet similar approaches: health persuasion, legislative action, personal counselling and community development.

Health persuasion is similar perhaps to a combination of health education and behavioural change. It is an intervention aimed at individuals and led by professionals. An example is a midwife encouraging a pregnant woman to stop smoking or a poster showing the negative effects of substance misuse on the body. Health persuasion will be discussed in more detail in later chapters.

Legislative actions are paternalistic or state-directed actions, such as making children travel in the back seat of cars and smoking bans. This equates to Ewles and Simnett's societal change approach, although Beattie by concentrating on legislative action ignores the myriad of society-wide agreements and policies which are in fact much more common than legislative action which in fact is quite rare. The passing of laws is serious business, hard to reverse and needs a great deal of public support and parliamentary time to enact.

Personal counselling represents client-led interventions and focuses on personal development. In this way, it matches the empowerment approach, with the health promoter acting as a facilitator rather than an expert. An example may be an alcohol support worker working with a client to identify their drinking patterns and with input from the client working together to draw up an action plan whose aim is to limit drinking to a level that the client feels he can manage to sustain. Personal counselling if done correctly is a time hungry approach, and before clients reach the stage of being able to embark on behaviour change, they may require in-depth and prolonged exploration of past experiences, learned behaviour patterns and efforts to increase self-confidence and self-efficacy. Without these in-depth interventions what can commonly happen is that messages and action plans are just laid over persistent problems and the client is doomed to fail, with the consequent decrease in self-belief which would inevitably accompany this. Personal counselling will be discussed in more detail in later chapters. Community development seeks to empower or enhance the skills of a group or local community. It facilitates community participation and involvement in addressing the needs of communities and can subsequently seek to tackle health inequalities. This may include the formation of neighbour groups to work on specific projects such as a food co-operative, a community garden or a toy library. Traditionally community development health promotion work has been focused on environmental issues and services, although it can be more clinically focused along the biomedical model.

Beattie's model uses the four quadrants between the two axes to illustrate how approaches interact with each other and how they are combined. If we take improving child road safety and preventing accidents, for example, as the aim of a series of interventions using different approaches, then Figure 4.2 illustrates the specific interventions that could be used in the relevant quadrant of the model. The quadrant between authoritative and individual which incorporates health persuasion could encompass local authority child accident statistics collected and given to the parents of children, hence raising awareness of the issue. The quadrant between authoritative and collective incorporating legislation could consist of an intervention to set a lower 20 miles an hour speed limit on roads near schools. The quadrant between collective to negotiated which incorporates community development could be working with the school community to organise walking buses, where volunteers walk children to school in groups. Setting up a group of interested parents in this way can lead to many interventions, for example, lobbying for speed bumps to slow traffic in the local vicinity. The quadrant between negotiated to individual incorporating personal counselling could include parents talking with their children about road safety.

Tones and Tilford's Empowerment Model of Health Promotion

The Tones and Tilford (2001) model suggests that health promotion is a combination of health education and healthy public policy. Policies aimed at promoting health will be discussed in more detail later; however, it is important here to define what is meant by healthy public policy. For this, it is useful to revisit Winslow's definition of public health in which he stated that public health interventions were brought about by 'the organised efforts of society' (Winslow 1923). Healthy public policy is just that, policies, systems, laws, agreements and ways of working put into place that seek to ensure that the health status of individuals and nations is improved. Policies are adopted which enhance health and very importantly policies are not implemented that contribute towards worsening health; therefore, all policies should enhance health and well-being. It can be argued, as has been seen in Chapter 1, that due to a wide range of health determinants, all policies have the potential to influence health. However, healthy public policy generally refers to social, environmental, political and economic measures as well as provision of health services and equity of access (Kemm 2001). Tones and Tilford state that health education is the root of all health promotion

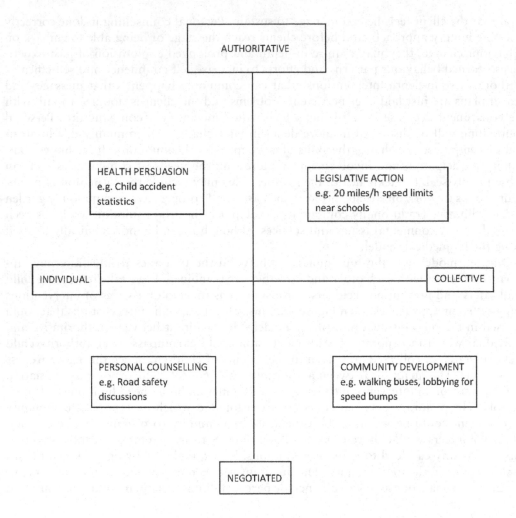

Figure 4.2 Beattie's (1991) Model Adapted to Show Ways of Addressing Child Road Safety

activities and hence they place health education at the bottom of their model with all other aspects growing upwards from it. Certainly, it is logical that knowledge of the influences on health is essential before changes will be made. Health education, they state, leads to awareness or critical conscious raising and the setting of agendas to improve health. They also make the leap from health education to the empowerment of individuals and communities; certainly health education needs to be in place, but there needs to be a lot of work before one naturally leads to the other. Empowerment leads both to the individual adopting a healthier lifestyle and communities lobbying for change. By talking of coalitions, they acknowledge the partnership working needed for effective health promotion, with local authorities, health services, community groups, voluntary organisations and business all working together towards similar goals. All the above they state form the bedrock on which healthy public policy is constructed and put into place, which in turn improves health. For local delivery of key policies and guidelines to be effective, it is essential that individuals and local communities are empowered and truly involved in decision-making and

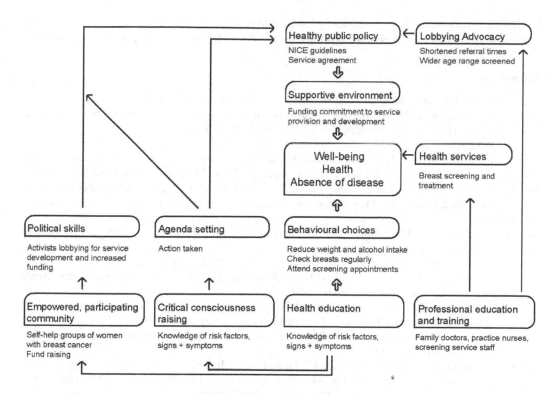

Figure 4.3 Adaptation of Tones and Tilford Model in Regard to Breast Cancer (2001)

implementation (Marmot 2010). Figure 4.3 illustrates how the model may be used with regard to breast cancer prevention and treatment.

By this stage, readers may be starting to identify familiar ways of working that they may have become involved in through their work as a health promoter. Nurses may recognise the medical and behavioural approaches and take part in these aspects, whereas a health promotion specialist may be more familiar with liaising with local community groups to assess their needs and help them with funding and resources to achieve agreed goals. A health information librarian will recognise their role in providing up-to-date health education material in the form of posters, leaflets, reports, books etc. both for professionals and the general public. A youth worker may be involved in working one to one with their clients on specific issues, but may also be a part of a wider group lobbying for change or resources for their client group. Whatever the specific role, it is essential to be able to understand the theory and reasons behind adopting certain interventions and also to consider the wider picture of how the public health workforce works together to instigate change.

Key Messages

- There are five main approaches to health promotion.
- Different approaches are used in combination to ensure effectiveness and impact.
- Models of health promotion illustrate how these approaches can work together in practice.
- Health promoters are encouraged to meet the specific agenda of their clients, although this is usually influenced and constrained by policies and funding.

- Health promoters adopt certain approaches and work within parameters according to their specific roles; however, all combine to produce effective health promotion practice.

References

Action on Smoking and Health. (2020). *Stopping smoking: The benefits and aids to quitting* [online]. Available at: https://ash.org.uk/information-and-resources/smoking-cessation-treatment/smoking-cessation/stopping-smoking-the-benefits-and-aids-to-quitting/

Baggott, R. (2010). *Public health policy and politic.* 2nd ed. Basingstoke: Palgrave Macmillan.

Baum, F. and Fisher, M. (2014). Why behavioural health promotion endures despite its failure to reduce health inequities *Sociology of Health & Illness*, 36(2), pp. 213–225. doi: 10.1111/1467-9566.12112.

Beattie, A. (1991). *Knowledge and control in health promotion: A test case for social policy and social theory.* In Gaber, J., Calman, M. and Bury, M. (eds.), *The sociology of the health service.* London: Routledge.

Deloitte Centre for Health Solutions. (2022). *Negating the gap: Preventing ill health and promoting healthy behaviours.* London. Deloitte.

Department of Health. (2008). *NHS stop smoking services & nicotine replacement therapy.* http://webarchive.nationalarchives.gov.uk/+/www.dh.gov.uk/en/Publichealth/Healthimprovement/Tobacco/Tobaccogeneralinformation/DH_4002192

Ewles, L. and Simnett, I. (2003). *Promoting health: A practical guide.* 5th ed. London: Balliere Tindall.

Johns Hopkins Coronavirus Resource Center. (2022). *Understanding vaccination progress by country - Johns Hopkins Coronavirus Resource Center* [online]. Available at: https://coronavirus.jhu.edu/vaccines/international

Kayser, L., Karnoe, A., Duminski, E., Somekh, D. and Vera-Muñoz, C. (2019). A new understanding of health related empowerment in the context of an active and healthy ageing. *BMC Health Services Research* [online], 19(1). Available at: https://bmchealthservres.biomedcentral.com/articles/10.1186/s12913-019-4082-5

Kemm, J. (2001). Health impact assessment: A tool for healthy public policy. *Health Promotion International*, 16(1), pp. 79–85. doi: 10.1093/heapro/16.1.79

Marmot, M. (2010). *Fair society, healthy lives, strategic review of health inequalities in England post 2010.* Institute of Health Inequity.

Marmot, M.G., Altman, D.G., Cameron, D. and Wilcox, M. (2013). *Independent UK Panel on Breast Cancer Screening: The benefits and harms of breast cancer screening: an...* [online]. ResearchGate. Available at: https://www.researchgate.net/publication/237070532_Independent_UK_Panel_on_Breast_Cancer_ScreeningThe_benefits_and_harms_of_breast_cancer_screening_an_independent_review_The_Lancet_380_1778-1786

Masters, R., Anwar, E., Collins, B., Cookson, R. and Capewell, S. (2017). Return on investment of public health interventions: A systematic review. *Journal of Epidemiology and Community Health* [online], 71(8), pp. 827–834. Available at: https://jech.bmj.com/content/71/8/827

National Institute for Health and Care Excellence (NICE). (2022). *What we do.* Available at: https://www.nice.org.uk/about/what-we-do

National Institute for Health Research Evidence. (2020). *Smoking bans improve cardiovascular health and reduce smoking-related deaths - NIHR Evidence* [online]. Available at: https://evidence.nihr.ac.uk/alert/smoking-bans-improve-cardiovascular-health-and-reduce-smoking-related-deaths/#:~:text=Thirty%2Dthree%20of%2043%20moderate,bans%20significantly%20reduced%20stroke%20rates.&text=Eight%20of%2011%20low%20quality,bans%20reduced%20smoking%2Drelated%20deaths

NHS Choices. (2022). *PSA testing - Prostate cancer* [online]. Available at: https://www.nhs.uk/conditions/prostate-cancer/psa-testing/

Office for National Statistics (ONS). (2021). *UK health accounts.* Available at: https://www.ons.gov.uk/peoplepopulationandcommunity/ healthandsocialcare/healthcaresystem/datasets/healthaccounts referencetables

Public Health England (PHE). (2019). *Public health strategy 2020-2025*. London. PHE.

Sathyanarayana Rao, T. and Andrade, C. (2011). The MMR vaccine and autism: Sensation, refutation, retraction, and fraud. *Indian Journal of Psychiatry* [online], 53(2), p. 95. Available at: https://www.ncbi.nlm.nih.gov/pmc/articles/PMC3136032/

Seely, J.M. and Alhassan, T. (2018). Screening for breast cancer in 2018—What should we be doing today? *Current Oncology* [online], 25(11), pp. 115–124. Available at: https://www.ncbi.nlm.nih.gov/pmc/articles/PMC6001765/

The King's Fund. (2021). *Integrated care systems explained making sense of systems, places and neighbourhoods* [online]. The King's Fund. Available at: https://www.kingsfund.org.uk/publications/integrated-care-systems-explained

Tones, K. and Tilford, S. (2001). *Health promotion effectiveness, efficiency, equity*. London: Nelson Thomas.

Torjesen, I. (2021). Measles outbreaks likely as covid pandemic leaves millions of world's children unvaccinated, WHO warns. *BMJ* [online], p. 2755. Available at: https://www.bmj.com/content/375/bmj

Whitehead, D. and Irvine, F. (2010). *Health promotion and health education in nursing*. Basingstoke: Palgrave Macmillan.

Winslow, C.E.A. (1923). *The evolution and significance of the modern public health campaign*. New Haven, CT. Yale University Press.

World Health Organization (WHO). (1986). *Ottawa Charter for health promotion: An international conference on health promotion*. Copenhagen: WHO.

World Health Organization (WHO). (2021). *Global progress against measles threatened amidst COVID-19 pandemic* [online]. Who.int. Available at: https://www.who.int/news/item/10-11-2021-global-progress-against-measles-threatened-amidst-covid-19-pandemic

World Health Organization (WHO). (n.d.). *Community empowerment*. Available at: https://www.who.int/teams/health-promotion/enhanced-wellbeing/seventh-global-conference/community-empowerment

5 Health Needs Assessment

Susan R. Thompson

Definition of Health Needs Assessment

Health needs assessment (HNA) has been described as 'a systematic method of identifying unmet health and healthcare needs of a population and making changes to meet these unmet needs' (Wright and Kyle 2006, p. 20) or 'Needs assessment is the collection and analysis of information that relates to the needs of affected populations and that will help determine gaps between an agreed standard and the current situation' (World Health Organization [WHO] n.d., p. 314). Whereas clinicians, doctors and nurses, etc. focus on individual patient needs assessment on a one-one basis, public health focuses on the health of populations. These populations may be geographically linked, those living in a certain city locality for instance or, alternatively, sections of a community, young people's health, health of pregnant women or the elderly. Public health also focuses on the needs of groups of people affected by specific health issues, such as diabetes, coronary heart disease or mental health problems. These three specific population groupings generally form the focus for health needs assessments of populations, whereas individual health needs assessments are performed by specific health care professionals with their client caseload. Health needs assessment within public health is used to set the policy agenda, plan services and target resources effectively to result in maximum health benefits for both individuals and populations. HNA is conducted at different levels – internationally, through the work of the WHO, nationally by government health departments, locally by hospital, primary care and local authority organisations right down to neighbourhood groups. Large-scale health needs assessments are carried out by statutory, voluntary, community and private sector organisations such as strategic groups within health and local authority services. Key agencies such as education, transport, local business, leisure, housing, the police and community representatives work together in partnership to agreed goals.

Needs assessments are conducted to collect quantitative and qualitative information which should inform plans to address specific local health needs (Flowers and Evans 2020). Key data pertaining to a specific population group or issue such as morbidity and mortality, demographics such as age and ethnic grouping, socio-economic status, existing services and risk factors are all types of information which may inform HNAs. Before HNAs are commenced, there must be a commitment to addressing a certain issue within a particular target group. It is irresponsible to start a HNA and consult with a client group unless it is expected that something of benefit for that group will come from it; consultation and involvement raise expectations which should in part be met (WHO n.d.). This may not be a brand new service provision; it may be a service development or alteration to better meet the needs of that group. It is essential, therefore, that key senior managers who can drive through change and direct resources are involved and fully 'on board'. Ideally, there should be a project lead

DOI: 10.4324/9781003411321-5

who will liaise and coordinate the involvement of key people, consult with the client group, write up the findings and propose an action plan. Consultation may involve meeting with key neighbourhood groups or support groups dealing with a specific issue or meeting with concerned individuals. Other client-based information can be used such as service evaluations and questionnaires. It is important to make consultation an ongoing process (Public Health England 2021). It should happen at the start of a project to gain an overview and continue at intervals once plans have been formulated and again when plans are in action. Evaluations can then be used to assess whether the initiative or service improvement is actually meeting the clients' needs (Naidoo and Wills 2016).

Critical Thinking

Do HNAs automatically lead to policy making?

Does a 'know – do' gap exist where research is carried out but recommendations are not put into practice?

What might get in the way of pursuing solutions?

Much of the academic debate around HNA centres on the identification of needs. At a very basic level, the definition of a need is 'the difference between an actual state and a goal' (Liss 1998, p. 9).

Types of Need

A widely recognised description of different types of need was developed by Bradshaw in 1972. He introduced his taxonomy of needs, stating that there were four basic types of need: normative, felt, expressed and comparative.

Normative Needs are those decided on by professionals, and data is analysed regarding the prevalence of certain conditions and whether or not the incidence of those conditions is increasing. Standards are set, for example, the normal blood pressure range. Those people who exceed this range are diagnosed as having high blood pressure and offered medication to lower their blood pressure. They are judged as having a recognisable need in this regard by parameters set by health professionals. Another example is the national UK breast screening programme. The decision to offer three yearly mammography to women over the age of 50 was arrived at by research weighing up the cost versus benefit analysis of offering this nationwide. Such large health initiatives are sanctioned by the government but others are decided upon and put into place by local health trusts, local authorities and other smaller providers of health and social care. Epidemiology and research provide an essential evidence base for ascertaining the normative needs and these are discussed in more detail below. Normative health needs based on data collection methods are relatively easy to ascertain, although by no means comprehensive with needs assessment often adopting a narrow disease approach (Watson 2002).

Felt Needs are discerned by asking clients or patients what their own perceived needs are. These may or may not match what professionals assess people's needs to be. For example, a 55-year-old woman may be unconcerned about her risk of breast cancer, but may state that she needs more respite care for the older relative she is caring for. In her opinion, this is the greater need for her at the present time. A study in 2018 showed that the commonest reasons people had for presenting at family doctors were coughs, indigestion, back pain, skin problems, headaches and anxiety (Finley et al. 2018). Generally, however, such symptoms are not identified as priorities formulated in national strategies. In an attempt to discern felt needs, the public is usually consulted before services commence and also when services are in place. Questions arise regarding consultations with the public for a proposed service or policy. Is it true consultation? Have people been involved from the beginning? Is it a service that they want? Or, are they being consulted as to the finer points of the service rather than the actual fundamental necessity or structuring of the service? Are people given enough information so that they are able to give informed comments? Who is being consulted with? Is it the vocal minority or is it those truly representative of the client group being targeted? Most consultation exercises seem to be one-off events regarding a specific issue, initiated by service providers, rather than the public, with the potential service provider setting the questions (Bennett 2018). There has also been criticism regarding the lack of training in the consultation process, either by those professionals initiating it or by members of the public taking part. Skills in communication, negotiation, compromise, understanding of group dynamics and conflict resolution are all essential skills for people asked to debate emotive issues such as health care, as well as information regarding the specific issue under debate. Felt needs may be better termed desires and the public are generally less well informed than professionals regarding the many different pressures on health resources or the level of risk or effectiveness of interventions proposed.

Expressed needs are identified by monitoring people's actions, using statistics regarding the uptake of services provided. The assumption is that if a service wasn't necessary, then it would not be used. For example, if women didn't attend mammography, there would be poor service uptake and questions would be asked, possibly resulting in closing the service down. However, this is a simplistic reading of the issue. People may turn up for screening because they are persuaded that they should do by friends and family or service publicity, health scares, fear and anxiety or being made to feel irresponsible if they don't. There are many reasons why people chose whether or not to attend (Rosenstock 2005). Access to services also needs to be considered, including the cost of the service provided. In 2017, a report estimated that 800 million people around the world spent 10 per cent of their household income on health care costs for existing illness and disease (World Bank and WHO 2017). Looking at this, it is easy to speculate that additional spending/taxation for preventative services might feel like an extra burden and get a lower priority. The use of health services also varies between different demographic groups, so it doesn't necessarily follow that services are meeting client needs.

Comparative need is the assessment of needs based on what is provided for similar populations elsewhere. This is about addressing equity in access to health care and ensuring equal provision for equal needs. For example, one area may have a project to provide support to teenage parents, but another area with a similar population of teenage parents does not have a project. This is inequality in health care provision. It must be stressed that health equity is not about providing the same service for everyone, but that those with greater or lesser needs should be treated proportionately (Angelis, Kanavos and Montibeller 2016). As we have already seen, much of the work of public health and the health care systems is concentrated on addressing comparative needs.

Value-Driven Needs Assessment

In an ideal world, all needs would be met; however, this is not possible as 'capacity to benefit is always greater than available resources' (Wright and Kyle 2006, p. 21). Health care needs expand over time. Difficult choices need to be made between fulfilling one need and denying another. Health economists compare costs and benefits and needs are prioritised on the basis of most in need and cost-effective care. This approach is termed value-based health competition in health care (VBHC), where values equate to the best value for money spent and competition means consumer (public and patients) wants and needs. This system has been adopted by most of western health care systems and has brought a market economy into health care sectors with various providers competing with each other to offer the best care at the lowest price in response to consumer demand (Groenewoud, Westert and Kremer 2019). There is much controversy as to whether a market economy is appropriate for health care systems and whether patients can act as true consumers, picking and choosing health care services. Certainly, the UK's NHS doesn't feel that way. Patients don't have a lot of choice where or who they go to for care. Other western nations often give patients more choice (Downie 2018; Fisher 2013).

This system of health care provision involves health care commissioners deciding on which services to purchase from service providers. Judgements are made regarding prioritisation and this is what causes controversy. As a society, there is no doubt that judgements are made regarding prioritisation of need, what might be seen as a need by one person may be seen as an indulgence by another. Needs assessment may be influenced by the organisational agenda, targets and individual professionals' own beliefs and values (Watson 2002). Many factors influence this perception of need, the quality of the information available regarding a particular issue, the media, the political and economic climate and the cost of interventions, lobbying by pressure groups and the values that exist in society (Angelis et al. 2016). Health needs assessment is a combination of epidemiological statistical evidence, economics regarding cost versus capacity to benefit and values held by society. The fact that assessment of needs is influenced by the value judgements of the person or organisation making the assessment is an emotive one, but value judgements are made when health care resources are scarce, and rationing of care exists in all health care systems. In the UK, the National Institute of Health and Care Excellence (NICE) recommends that women under 40 should be entitled to three cycles of in vitro fertilisation (IVF) treatment (Nice.org.uk 2013), but a study in 2020 showed that only 23 out the 108 clinical commissioning groups offered three cycles of IVF, most only offering one cycle as other things are prioritised (British Pregnancy Advisory Service 2020).

Activity

Imagine that you are in the position to decide on health care funding for specific issues or individuals. Below are listed seven separate requests for funding that you have received. Unfortunately, you do not possess the resources to fund all of these, so you must choose two.

1 Coronary artery bypass graft for a 72-year-old woman with angina to stop her condition from worsening and possibly causing a heart attack.
2 Nicotine replacement therapy (NRT) or E cigarettes – free NRT or E cigarettes to those on low incomes to help them quit smoking.
3 Liver transplant for a 57-year-old man with alcoholic liver disease who says he is determined not to drink alcohol anymore.
4 Breastfeeding peer support programme – continuation of this programme which has evaluated well and increased the uptake of breastfeeding in the local community.

5 Routine inguinal hernia operation for a 36-year-old, otherwise a fit man.
6 Chemotherapy for a 9-year-old boy with leukaemia which might possibly cure him.
7 Occupational therapy – funding for an Occupational Therapist to work with adults with learning disabilities to increase their independence.

In order to decide on which two to fund, you may wish to perform quick searches to understand the conditions/interventions in brief. Things you may consider are: the age of the individual/s, the benefit (economic or otherwise) to society, the severity of the issue, the chance of full recovery/success, long-term versus short-term gains and whether they are deserving of care.

Decision-Makers

Decisions regarding priorities for funding specific services or interventions, clinical or otherwise, take place on a regular basis within health care bodies. In England, Integrated Care Partnerships are a broad alliance of local organisations that come together to plan and commission hospital, community and mental health and family doctor services, and also social care and well-being services. Such local partnerships consist of health and local authority services, voluntary institutions, local residents and service users (NHS England 2022). The bringing together of social care with health services follows a model that was adopted in Scotland in 2016, with the aim of a seamless transition of patients between health and social care services, a major challenge in recent years (Scottish Government 2016). Local authorities have the health improvement/health promotion remit for their locality running, for example, quit smoking services, sexual health services and the myriad of different health promotion initiatives and projects which tackle different health determinants. Integrated Care Partnerships (ICPs) came into operation in England in 2022 and at the time of writing, it is envisaged that health needs assessment at a local 'place' level will still be enacted by Health and Well Being Boards. These are tasked with performing a Joint Strategic Needs Assessment (JSNA) which will feed into ICPs to determine future actions and priorities (Local.gov.uk 2020; NHS England 2022).

The decision to shift the responsibility of health promotion services from NHS primary care trusts to local authorities was seen as a good move in 2013 as very often health promotion services suffered from being part of the NHS, which is heavily focused on diagnosis and treatment of health conditions and less driven by preventative care. As we have seen, a significant number of health determinants are social and environmental and the local authorities with its remit for providing leisure services, parks and gardens, cycle paths, street lighting, community centres, youth centres, educational provision, housing, play centres and transport, etc., have the potential to have a significant impact on these determinants. Commonly in the NHS, health promotion budgets were raided to pay for overspending in other areas such as medication and to reduce waiting times for surgical procedures (Baggott 2000; Entwhistle, Darlow and Downe 2007). Unfortunately, the move to local authorities coincided with substantial funding cuts to these bodies which affected all areas of responsibility including public health (National Audit Office 2018). The King's Fund estimates that the public health grant to local government would be 24% lower in real terms in 2021/2022 than it was in 2015/2016 (The King's Fund 2019). Funding cuts to public health are a false economy, only storing up health care problems in the future which will need expensive in-patient or community care (Masters et al. 2017). There are signs already filtering through that such cuts are leading to worrying trends in population health (Alexiou, Fahy and Mason 2021; Lewer and Bibby 2021).

Effective Interventions

Any HNA should also incorporate an assessment of interventions proposed, their effectiveness and cost-effectiveness. Systematic reviews of interventions used to target specific issues are published in the UK by The Cochrane Library and NICE. These reviews take individual pieces of research on specific interventions published in academic journals and analyse them for rigour. A conclusion is then drawn on their effectiveness and recommendations made. Health needs assessment is the first stage in public health or health promotion programme planning and this programme evaluation forms the focus of a later chapter.

Health needs assessment should use a combination of information sources in order to obtain a clear picture of the issues for the population concerned. Epidemiological sources of information are available in the form of statistics and research, for example, disease rates. This approach is discussed in more detail below. Information then needs to be sought from agencies and organisations regularly in contact with the population group, for example, the range of existing service providers. The felt needs of the population or community under question need to be sought to gain information on priorities for that population, what is thought about existing services, what could be improved and what is needed instead (Davies and Macdowall 2006; Whitehead and Irvine 2010). It is important to remember that HNAs can be used to assess a range of services and interventions, not just clinical services, but also community projects and rehabilitation and support services.

Epidemiology

Simply put, epidemiology can be defined as the study of how often diseases reoccur in different groups of people and why (BMJ 2020). Epidemiology, therefore, studies the causes of disease and disease distribution patterns. From this, advice can be given to policy makers on potential interventions in order to prevent or reduce exposure of the population to these causations and public policy formulated to reduce the exposure. The birth of the modern public health movement probably began with the Victorian pioneer, John Snow. Snow had been researching outbreaks of cholera in London for some time, trying to establish the cause of these, when, in 1854, a serious outbreak occurred in Soho. At that time, many physicians and academics thought that smells and foul air transmitted disease. This was termed the miasma theory. However, Snow believed in germ theory, that microorganisms, lately discovered by Pasteur, spread infectious disease. Snow coloured in a map of the houses in the locality where people lived who had been affected by cholera and found out that all the people affected drew their water from one particular street pump. He took the handle off the pump and stopped the epidemic. The experiment then needed repeating in another location with cholera in order to categorically prove the association. This discovery of the absolute need for a clean, non-contaminated water supply and an efficient sewage system caused the development of London's sewage system and, consequently, the separation of waste from the water supply, which became a model for other cities worldwide (Porter 1999). In the following century, public health concentrated mainly on improving environmental conditions, for example, preventing overcrowding, improving sanitation and clearing slum housing to help prevent spread of infectious disease (Rees 2001). At the time of his experiment, Snow was unsure of the organism causing the cholera outbreak; however, in judging the water to be at fault and then stopping that water from being used, he established a fundamental principle of epidemiology. He formulated a hypothesis (contaminated water) and tested it (by removing the pump handle), thus endeavouring to prove causation. In the modern world, the gathering of information regarding possible causes of disease, such as examining distribution patterns and determining factors in common, and then the experimental testing of interventions are essential components in both medicine and public health. However, it is still the case that for many conditions the actual mechanism, whereby certain factors cause disease, is largely unknown. There have been many studies about sudden infant death syndrome; for example, it is now generally accepted that certain factors increase this risk. Sudden infant death syndrome is more likely in babies under four months of age, of low birth weight and those born to mothers under 20 years of age. Sudden infant deaths are associated with babies becoming overheated and babies being placed on their front or side to sleep and are more common in households that smoke and more deaths occur in winter. Protective factors that have been shown to reduce the risk of these deaths are breastfeeding and use of dummies (Lullabytrust.org.uk 2021). Nevertheless, although these causal factors have been established, why these factors cause cot deaths is still uncertain. This is not uncommon in the field of public health. Evidence is accumulated as to possible causes and effects and further research is undertaken. Meanwhile, people are advised of these possible links. In the 1950s, a revolutionary study proved the link between smoking and lung cancer by studying tobacco use and rates of lung cancer in smokers and non-smokers (Doll and Hill 1950). This, like all good public health research, led to informed public policy, although in the case of smoking, the commonality of this behaviour and the political ramifications associated with tobacco control meant that many years went by before effective governmental measures were put in place targeted at reducing smoking levels in the population.

Epidemiological Data

In the modern era, epidemiology has access to a range of statistical sources which can contribute to health needs assessment. There are census data, hospital admission rates, cancer registers, index of multiple deprivations scores, employment statistics, surgical operations data, ethnic origin data, emergency department admissions and notifiable diseases registers, to name but a few. Three fundamental measures that are used by public health specialists to chart the course and scope of disease are prevalence and incidence rates and standardised mortality ratios. Prevalence is the proportion of the population which has a disease or condition at a particular point in time (Robinson and Elkan 1996), for example, the percentage of Sheffield's population who are undergoing renal dialysis for chronic renal failure in Sheffield hospitals at the present time. Incidence rates deal with new cases (Robinson and Elkan 1996), for example, the number of women in the UK who were newly diagnosed as having multiple sclerosis in 2021. Potential incidence statistics can be expressed as people at risk of developing a certain condition. For example, if an originally healthy population of a 100 is followed for a year, 10 people may, at the end of that year, have been found to have developed arthritis. Therefore, the risk of developing arthritis in a year within that population studied was found to be 0.1 or 10%. Statistics in epidemiology are of little use unless they are compared with statistics from other areas or population groups. Otherwise, how would you know that Sheffield has more or less chronic renal failure cases than elsewhere? Also, it depends on the population studied. Arthritis is a disease common in the elderly. Therefore, a study of 20-year-olds will naturally give different results compared with a study of 70-year-olds. Standardised mortality ratios (SMRs) are used to even up this discrepancy seen in populations so that a true comparison can be made. SMRs compare the actual death rate in a specific population with the expected death rate in that population, taking into account the different demographics of that particular population. The standard expected death rate is put at a 100. Therefore, populations that have SMRs over a 100 have a higher death rate than expected and those with SMRs below a 100 have a lower than expected death rate. This is obviously incremental; for example, a geographical area with a SMR of 50 for breast cancer has half the risk of its women developing breast cancer than the national average. Usually, the data is age adjusted, so the differences in the age demographics are taken into account. However, there are many other variables which are different in different population groups, gender, ethnic origin and social economic status, for instance, all of which as we have seen have an influence on disease. It is difficult to account for all these variables. Therefore, a true comparison cannot be made and SMRs remain a blunt instrument, if a useful indicator. It is to be stressed that SMRs deal in death only, so incidence and prevalence rates are very important in considering other conditions or issues. Incidence rates are particularly useful for conditions which are short in duration or acute episodes, infectious diseases for example, whereas prevalence rates are most useful for long-term chronic conditions such as diabetes and asthma. Epidemiological research studies investigate possible factors or determinants which may cause disease. The four common study designs are cross sectional studies, case control studies, cohort studies and intervention studies. A brief introduction to each of them is given below.

Cross Sectional Studies

Cross sectional studies or prevalence studies are one-off, snapshot studies. They divide a population into two and look at a specific factor in relation to the two groups, for example, age of menopause and coronary heart disease in women. One group may be those who reached their menopause before the age of 55 years and the other group after 55. Rates of CHD for both groups are then accessed and a possible link is discovered, for example, women who had earlier menopause have a greater risk of CHD. Of course, this doesn't necessarily prove cause and effect, and there may be many other unknown factors which link the women who developed CHD, but it is the start to take the research further.

Cohort Studies

Cohort or longitudinal studies are prospective. A large group of healthy people are selected, and data is taken from them at the start. Throughout the study period, they are followed for a number of years and the results in respect of the development of certain conditions are analysed and links made between the development of certain condition and factors common to those in the cohort who developed this condition. There are many studies using this design. In the UK, the Breakthrough Generations study seeks to discover the causes of breast cancer by following 100,000 UK women over a 40-year period (Breakthroughgenerations. org.uk 2022). There is also the Millennium Cohort Study which is following around 20,000 UK children born at the turn of the century. As cohort studies progress, initial findings are discovered. In 2021, findings were already showing that this cohort of young people is showing high levels of psychological distress and self-harm, that a third of them are either overweight or obese and that 10% had already tried 'hard drugs' (University College London 2021). Both cross sectional and cohort studies rely on the recruitment of a substantial number of people in order to show up enough results to be statistically significant. They also need to study conditions which are quite commonplace, as if conditions are rare there may be too few in the sample group to draw any conclusions from.

Case Control Studies

Case control studies are retrospective. They select study participants all of whom have a particular disease or condition and then compare them for certain factors such as level of alcohol intake, smoking status, etc. These are then compared to a group who do not have that condition and the differences in behaviour or other factors are noted. Case control studies can also be used to assess the success of interventions, for example, what might be the benefit or not for those patients who receive cardiac rehabilitation after a heart attack compared to those who did not. Case control studies examine factors retrospectively. What was the intervention or factors? What was the result? As case control studies start with people already diagnosed with the condition under scrutiny, fewer numbers can be used and rarer conditions studied.

Experimental Studies

The final category of study is the intervention or experimental study in which a matched population (one that has as many commonalities as possible, e.g. age group, gender, etc.) is divided into two, with half being given an intervention and half not. This is commonly used in drug treatments. A randomised controlled trial (RCT) is considered an excellent study design, especially if it is double blinded. In double blind trials, placebos are used for the group who does not receive an intervention and neither the participant nor the staff administering the intervention are aware which participant receives what. RCTs are easier for drug treatments. It is more difficult to assess whether physical activity, for example, improves mood. After all, people will know whether they are doing physical activity or not, and it cannot be hidden from them. Researchers may, however, be able to divide the group into those doing recommended levels or types of physical activity and those not. There are many issues that can occur with research such as errors in sampling, bias and confounding which are beyond the remit of this book. However, epidemiological research and statistics and also qualitative research form an important evidence base for health needs assessment if they are analysed properly.

Risk Assessment

Risks are the association of various factors with the probability of contracting disease or conditions. For example, driving too fast puts people more at risk of an accident and smoking puts them more at risk of lung cancer. More research is still needed to understand the mechanisms involved as although the cause and effect may be proven, much is still unknown. For example, strong personal relationships have been proved to be a protective factor in reducing morbidity and delayed mortality, but why this is the case is still largely a matter of conjecture.

Activity Answers

There are no definitive answers to this activity. What is important is the analysis of the decision-making process. What was the thinking behind the choice of your top two most deserving cases? Given below is a possible summary of the factors that you may have taken into account when making your decision.

Inguinal Hernia Repair: Usually a straightforward surgical procedure with a high chance of success without complications, relatively cheap with a long-term cure probable. The person is young and, therefore, has ahead of him a long active life during which he will, if fit, be able to contribute positively to society, both economically and socially. However, unless complications arise, this is not a life-threatening issue and men can live for years with a hernia like this without it significantly affecting their lives.

Liver Transplant: Providing a liver transplant to someone who has damaged their liver through excessive drinking will possibly raise public concerns that the patient is undeserving of resources due to the perceived self-inflicted nature of the problem, although this could be said about many health issues. Does the stigma associated with alcohol addiction generate more public censure than other health complaints? The man has given up drinking and if he maintains this, the prognosis should be good, but can he 'be trusted' to maintain his abstinence? What support may be available to help him with this?

Peer Support Breastfeeding: Breastfeeding has been linked to long-term health gains, from an increase in intelligence to reduced infection rates and a decrease in allergies. This intervention has been evaluated well so appears to be working therefore has a proven track record. Children are the main beneficiaries of this work and many people can be reached by this intervention. However, children do manage perfectly well by being bottle fed. So, how necessary is this intervention?

Coronary Artery Bypass Graft Surgery: This procedure is usually successful in alleviating blockages in the arteries supplying the heart, therefore reducing significantly the risk of the patient having a heart attack and also relieving the patient's angina pain. However, this procedure is fairly expensive. As the patient is already 72, how much productive life has she got left and due to her age isn't she just going to get another health issue? Can medication be used instead which will provide quality of life?

Chemotherapy: The recipient of care here is a young boy. Society tends to prioritise care for children as they are seen as blameless, having their whole life ahead of them and it being unfair to have it prematurely taken from them. Society emotionally invests in its children to a significant degree. However, chemotherapy can be quite expensive and is it actually going to work? Often, chemotherapy only prolongs life for a period of time, will it cure?

Free Nicotine Replacement Therapy and/or E Cigarettes: Quitting smoking results in significant long-term health benefits to the individual and reduces costs to society in treating diseases linked to smoking. Therefore, isn't funding this a good investment? Alternatively, it's the smokers who have decided to smoke, so shouldn't they pay for their own medication with the money they will save from not smoking? Also, many smokers start smoking again, so isn't free treatment a waste of money?

Occupational Therapy for Adults with Learning Disabilities: Adults with learning disabilities can gain a better quality of life and be less dependent on services, family and carers if they are supported in learning life skills. One OT can work with many people, so isn't this cost-effective? However, how much change can really be made? Will this client group ever be able to get jobs and contribute to society?

The discussions above are simplistic and the questions posed played devil's advocate and could possibly be considered offensive in some cases. The aim is to show a little of the value judgements that are made by society when deciding on who deserves scarce resources. Value judgements are made blatantly in the case of welfare benefit recipients. Any vox pop poll by reporters in the street shows this. People may be more reticent to express their opinions in the area of health care, but judgements are still made, even if just privately. There is also evidence of a tug of war between the social model of health which is often more to do with improving people's lives and the medical model of health which often prioritises cure and medical interventions over social interventions.

Key Messages

- Health needs assessments vary in scale, can be conducted by a range of different agencies and are used to set the policy agenda, plan services and target resources effectively.
- There are different types of need but often normative needs take precedence when undertaking health needs assessment.
- Epidemiology plays an important part in informing health needs assessment. Disease incidence and prevalence rates can be charted and risk and protective factors associated with certain health issues can be identified.
- Although health needs assessments often originate from departments of health and national priorities, it is important to consult with the target group and people working with that group in order to prioritise goals and gain feedback on ways of working.
- Value judgements are made when deciding on access to health care and public health services. Decision-makers may be influenced by powerful advocates for particular aspects of care, by public perceptions of priorities in care, by cost-effectiveness of interventions and short- and long-term goals and targets.

References

Alexiou, A., Fahy, K. and Mason, K. (2021). Local government funding and life expectancy in England: A longitudinal ecological study. *Lancet Public Health*. https://doi.org/10.1016/S2468-2667(21)00110-9

Angelis, A., Kanavos, P. and Montibeller, G. (2016). Resource allocation and priority setting in health care: A multi-criteria decision analysis problem of value? *Global Policy* [online], 8, pp. 76–83. Available at: https://onlinelibrary.wiley.com/doi/full/10.1111/1758-5899.12387

Baggott, R. (2000). *Public health policy and politics*. Basingstoke: Palgrave Macmillan.

Bennett, D. (2018). Public consultation in healthcare provision: The good, the bad and the unacceptable. *PharmaTimes* [online]. Available at: https://www.pharmatimes.com/web_exclusives/public_consultation_in_healthcare_provision_the_good,_the_bad_and_the_unacceptable_1237968

BMJ. (2020). Chapter 1. What is epidemiology? | *BMJ* [online]. Available at: https://www.bmj.com/about-bmj/resources-readers/publications/epidemiology-uninitiated/1-what-epidemiology

Bradshaw, J.R. (1972). The taxonomy of social need. In: McLachlan, G., ed. *Problems and progress in medical care*. Oxford: Oxford University Press.

Breakthroughgenerations.org.uk. (2022). Home | Generations Study [online]. Available at: https://www.breakthroughgenerations.org.uk/home

British Pregnancy Advisory Service. (2020). *Investigation into the IVF postcode lottery: An examination of CCG policy for the provision of fertility services* [online]. Available at: https://www.bpas.org/media/3369/bpas-fertility-ivf-postcode-lottery-report.pdf

Davies, M. and Macdowall, W. (2006). Planning a health promotion intervention. In *Health promotion theory*. Maidenhead: Open University Press.

Doll, R. and Hill, A.B. (1950). Smoking and carcinoma of the lung. *British Medical Journal*, 221(ii), pp. 739–48.

Downie, R. (2018). Patients and consumers. *Journal of the Royal College of Physicians of Edinburgh*, 47(3), pp. 261–265.

Entwhistle, T., Darlow, A. and Downe, J. (2007). *Perspectives on place shaping and service delivery*. Cardiff: Centre for regional and local government and research, Cardiff University.

Finley, C.R., Chan, D.S., Garrison, S., Korownyk, C., Kolber, M.R., Campbell, S., Eurich, D.T., Lindblad, A.J., Vandermeer, B. and Allan, G.M. (2018). What are the most common conditions in primary care? Systematic review. *Canadian family physician Medecin de famille canadien* [online], 64(11), pp. 832–840. Available at: https://www.ncbi.nlm.nih.gov/pmc/articles/PMC6234945/

Fisher, B. (2013). *The dangers of marketisation* [online]. Health Service Journal. Available at: https://www.hsj.co.uk/comment/the-dangers-of-marketisation-/5053782.article#:~:text=There%20are%20theoretical%20reasons%20why,and%20price%20signals%20working%20poorly

Flowers, J. and Evans, S. (2020). Assessing the health of populations. In: Kawachi, I., Lang, I. and Ricciardi, W., eds. *Oxford Handbook of public health practice*. 4th ed. Oxford: Oxford University Press.

Groenewoud, A.S., Westert, G.P. and Kremer, J.A.M. (2019). Value based competition in health care's ethical drawbacks and the need for a values-driven approach. *BMC Health Services Research* [online], 19(1). Available at: https://bmchealthservres.biomedcentral.com/articles/10.1186/s12913-019-4081-6

Lewer, D. and Bibby, J. (2021). Cuts to local government funding and stalling life expectancy. *The Lancet Public Health* [online], 6(9), pp. e623–e624. Available at: https://www.thelancet.com/journals/lanpub/article/PIIS2468-2667(21)00136-5/fulltext

Liss, P.E. (1998). Assessing health care need: The conceptual foundation. In: Baldwin, S., ed. *Needs assessment and community care*. Oxford: Butterworth-Heinemann, pp. 9–23.

Local.gov.uk. (2020). *Health and wellbeing systems* [online]. Available at: https://www.local.gov.uk/our-support/sector-support-offer/care-and-health-improvement/health-and-wellbeing-systems#:~:text=Health%20and%20Wellbeing%20Boards%20(HWBs,population%20and%20reduce%20health%20inequalities.&text=portfolio%2Dholders%2Flead%20members%20for%20public%20health

Lullabytrust.org.uk. (2021). *How to reduce the risk of SIDS for your baby* [online]. Available at: https://www.lullabytrust.org.uk/safer-sleep-advice/

Masters, R., Anwar, E., Collins, B., Cookson, C. and Capewell, S. (2017). Return on investment of public health interventions: A systematic review. *Journal Epidemiology and Community Health*, 71, pp. 827–834. doi: 10.1136/jech-2016-208141.

Naidoo, J. and Wills, J. (2016). *Foundations for health promotion*. 4th ed. London: Elsevier.

National Audit Office. (2018). *Financial sustainability of local authorities*. Available at: https://www.nao.org.uk/wp-content/uploads/2018/03/Financial-sustainabilty-of-local-authorites-2018.pdf

NHS England. (2022). *What are integrated care systems*. https://www.england.nhs.uk/integratedcare/what-is-integrated-care/

Nice.org.uk. (2013). *In vitro fertilisation | Information for the public | Fertility problems: assessment and treatment | Guidance | NICE* [online]. Available at: https://www.nice.org.uk/guidance/cg156/ifp/chapter/in-vitro-fertilisation

Porter, R. (1999). *The greatest benefit to mankind: A medical history of humanity from antiquity to the present*. London: Harper Collins.

Public Health England. (2021). *Population health needs assessment: A guide for 0 to 19 health visiting and school nursing services* [online]. GOV.UK. Available at: https://www.gov.uk/government/publications/commissioning-of-public-health-services-for-children/population-health-needs-assessment-a-guide-for-0-to-19-health-visiting-and-school-nursing-services

Rees, R. (2001). *Poverty and public health*. Oxford: Heineman.

Robinson, J. and Elkan, R. (1996). *Health needs assessment theory and practice*. New York: Churchill Livingstone.

Rosenstock, I.M. (2005). Why people use health services. *Milbank Quarterly* [online], 83(4). Available at: https://www.ncbi.nlm.nih.gov/pmc/articles/PMC2690262/

Scottish Government. (2016). *Health and social care integration.* https://www.gov.scot/policies/social-care/health-and-social-care-integration/

The King's Fund. (2019). *Public health: Our position* [online]. Available at: https://www.kingsfund.org.uk/projects/positions/public-health

University College London. (2021). *Initial findings from the Millennium Cohort Study Age 17 Sweep* [online]. Available at: https://cls.ucl.ac.uk/cls_research/initial-findings-from-the-millennium-cohort-study-age-17-survey/

Watson, M. (2002). Normative needs assessment: Is this an appropriate way in which to meet the new public health agenda. *International Journal of Health Promotion and Education*, 40(1), pp. 4–8.

Whitehead, D. and Irvine, F. (2010). *Health promotion and health education in nursing.* Basingstoke: Palgrave Macmillan.

World Bank and WHO. (2017). *Half the world lacks access to essential health services, 100 million still pushed into extreme poverty because of health expenses.* Available at: https://www.who.int/news/item/13-12-2017-world-bank-and-who-half-the-world-lacks-access-to-essential-health-services-100-million-still-pushed-into-extreme-poverty-because-of-health-expenses

World Health Organization. (n.d.) *Needs assessment.* Available at: https://www.who.int/health-cluster/resources/publications/hc-guide/HC-Guide-chapter-10.pdf?ua=1

Wright, J. and Kyle, D. (2006). Assessing health needs. In: Pencheon, D., Guest, G., Melzer, D. and Muir Grey, J.A., eds. *Oxford Handbook of public health practice.* Oxford: Oxford University Press.

6   Health Education and Information

Susan R. Thompson

Health education is the combination of learning experiences, development of life skills and health literacy designed to help individuals and communities improve their health by increasing their knowledge or influencing their attitudes. Health education is an essential first step for health promotion. After all, unless people are aware of the cause and effect, that smoking cigarettes, for example, significantly increases the risk of developing lung cancer, why should they think about quitting? During the last century, knowledge of the causes of ill health increased dramatically and this led to resources being directed towards the education of the public regarding a multitude of risk factors and the part they play in a range of diseases. The widespread improvement in living conditions and the presence of antibiotic and antiviral therapy have in the developed world at least reduced the number, severity and spread of infections. This has caused public health to focus on chronic long-term health conditions which affect longevity and quality of life and are linked to behavioural factors. Much of the work of health educators, therefore, is around informing people of the nature of these risk factors and helping people with behaviour change. However, health education is not just focused on helping people avoid the risk factors associated with chronic conditions, but health educators also tackle issues such as sexual health, teenage pregnancy, road safety and mental well-being, for instance.

Health Literacy

It is important to note that in order for people to take on board health promotion messages, they need to be able to fully understand those messages. In the narrowest sense, being health literate means being able to understand medicine leaflets, follow self-care instructions and appreciate the causes of ill health. On a broader level, being health literate enables people to engage with their own health and communicate effectively with health care providers and navigate health care systems and allows them to make informed decisions and understand and act on health messages. Low health literacy has been associated with failing to adopt healthier behaviours, less health self-management and consequently poorer health status (WHO 2019). There has been much debate around the levels of health literacy in the general population with studies showing that health information is very often presented in an inaccessible format and presumes an educational level in excess of that of the educational level of much of the population (Keçeci, Toprak and Kiliç 2017; Maskell, McDonald and Paudyal 2018). Tables and graphs often present in health information resources further compound this inaccessibility. It also follows that information which goes above the head of the general population will be even more inaccessible for those who do not have the native tongue as their first language or for those with a degree of learning disability. Research has

DOI: 10.4324/9781003411321-6

shown that the use of symbols and illustrations rather than blank text can significantly increase comprehension (Jungmin and Zuniga 2016). Client involvement in the development of materials has also proven to be effective, as has the use of videos, animated cartoons and computer interactive software (Leiner, Handel and Williams et al. 2004; Meade, McKinney and Barnas 1994; Rudd and Comings 1994). Much health information reaches us via digital sources but the unregulated nature of these sources means that much on the internet is of dubious quality, making it even more important that people are able to navigate to reputable sources of information (Battineni et al. 2020; Griebel et al. 2017).

The Limits of Health Information

It is a fallacy to think that merely informing people of the risks and benefits of certain behaviour results in behaviour change. Health knowledge in developed societies is perhaps greater than ever before, but preventable health issues stubbornly persist. The majority of public health policies still centre around providing such information; however, health education is just one strand in the process towards behaviour change and on its own is relatively ineffective. Individual behaviour is complex and society's influences on this behaviour are very pervasive (Becker 1999). Health promotion campaigns do have the potential to change attitudes and increase knowledge of certain issues, especially tobacco control (Kuipers et al. 2017; Sims et al. 2014), although evidence of effectiveness for other issues remains limited (National Institute Health and Care Research (NIHR) Evidence 2019). The job of campaigns is to raise awareness of an issue and point people in the direction of services to provide further support. Health information is often targeted at patients attending family doctor or hospital appointments in the form of posters or leaflets. Studies have shown that although posters are read, recall of their content after some time has elapsed is very limited (Maskell et al. 2018; Ward and Hawthorne 1994; Wicke et al. 1994). Nevertheless, there has been some success with using posters as prompts. One project showed that posters positioned in stairwells and lift lobbies were effective at prompting people to use the stairs instead of the lift (Kerr, Eves and Carroll 2000). This was possibly because the message conveyed was simple and easy to activate with immediate effect. It is well recognised that interactive teaching techniques are much more effective than passive ones (Benware 1984; Kolb 1984). Digital resources benefit from being interactive. Although incorporating smarter digital technology brings health promotion and public health interventions into the modern age, actually the result is the same. The emphasis is still on personal responsibility and what individuals should be doing.

Advertising and the Art of Persuasion

In his book *Brave New World*, Aldous Huxley wrote 'find some common desire, some widespread unconscious fear or anxiety; think of some way to relate this wish or fear to the product you have to sell; then build a bridge from the dream to the illusion that your product, when purchased, will make the dream come true' (Huxley 1932). This is the way advertisers sell products; for example, a fear of growing and looking old may result in the production of anti-aging creams, and advertisers then persuade older women that their product will make them look younger. A common desire to be free could be exploited by advertisers of new cars with television images of convertibles driving along deserted mountain roads and alongside waterfalls, giving the impression that with this car your dream will be realised. Advertisers don't place their cars in traffic jams. In the modern world, the public is bombarded with health messages from a range of sources. This involves the art of persuasion, and in recent years health promoters have sought the expertise of the advertising industry to compile media campaigns which aim to connect with a target group, get the message across and hopefully achieve behaviour change. The ability to connect with the audience is essential; target audiences need to be able to relate to the central character in a TV advert or a social media post, for example, and material needs to be accessible and engaging. The internet cannot be trusted as an unbiased source of information; for instance, researchers have shown that customer reviews are routinely manipulated in order to secure higher sales (David and Pinch 2006; Hu et al. 2009). Nevertheless, social media, and the internet in general, is an excellent and inexpensive tool for providing health education to a wide audience.

Corporations spend far more money on advertising their products than health organisations do trying to persuade people to adopt healthier behaviours. Governments try and redress some of this balance by working with industries to limit the power of advertising unhealthy behaviours. Cigarettes advertising was banned many years ago in the UK; however, advertisers find a way around such bans. Tobacco companies now produce adverts which use well-known iconography associated with known brands of cigarettes, packaging colours, hints at brand names, etc. to keep the brand in the public eye without having to even mention or show cigarettes. Governments are increasingly concerned with rising levels of obesity but food and drink manufacturers are a very powerful body and resist each proposed restriction. In October 2022, the UK banned in-store promotions of high fat, sugar and salty food (GOV. UK 2021). However, plans to ban fast food advertisements aimed at children were defeated. During the negotiations over the 2018 UK soft drink industry levy (commonly known as the sugar tax) which taxes high sugar soft drinks, the inclusion of certain products was contested by the industry, thereby slowing down the progress of the bill into law. This tax has proven successful, and the amount of sugar in soft drinks had reduced by 10% or 30 grams per household by 2019 (MRC Epidemiology Unit 2021). The next battleground may be sports sponsorship. At the moment, a famous chocolate brand sponsors a top English Premier League football club (Samadi 2023), with a very famous soft drink manufacturer sponsoring the Olympic Games consistently since 1928. Manufacturers must feel that this sponsorship is worthwhile and that they get a good return on their investment as they continue with such tactics and resist any controls placed on them.

Social Marketing

One way in which health promoters seek to alter attitudes and behaviour is through the social marketing approach which treats the public as potential consumers of health information and targets them using the principles and working practices established in the advertising industry. The approach seeks to influence audience behaviour that benefits society as well as the target audience (Kotler and Lee 2008), and basically social marketers sell behaviours. The aim is for people to make one of four behaviour changes – to *accept* (or adopt) a positive behaviour, for example, taking up jogging; to *reject* the adoption of a detrimental behaviour choice, for example, decide that they will not start smoking; *modify* an existing behaviour, for example, cut down their alcohol intake; and *abandon* completely a detrimental health behaviour, for example, quitting smoking (Cheng, Kotler and Lee 2009). Social marketing has brought the advertisers' knowledge of the human psyche to the forefront of health promotion and public health education. Essential to the social marketing campaign model is audience research (Kotler and Lee 2008). Once the target group is identified, an analysis of that audience, their desires, what makes them tick and what will capture their attention and help them to engage with the message is determined. Focus groups, surveys and psychological profiling either online or in person can help with this and draft campaign materials can be created and piloted with the help of volunteers from that audience. Key aspects for success in composing messages include presenting credible evidence from a credible source, making the message clear, using incentives, suggesting easy actions and interestingly placing the critical or most important aspect at the start of the message (Nccmt.ca. 2013). Research has been conducted into the effectiveness of social marketing for health promotion and public health and some success in behaviour change is evident (Firestone et al. 2017).

The Hard Sell

The difficulty with having access to the wealth of information we are bombarded with is that people can suffer from information overload and just switch off. Advertisers, therefore, need to create items that capture attention, to stand out from the crowd, and this has led to more sensationalist practices so that messages can be noticed in the noise of other outlets. This results in hard-hitting campaigns with a tendency to present messages negatively, that is, 'if you don't do this (or don't stop doing that), something awful will happen to you'. The UK along with Australia, Canada and some other countries now requires manufacturers of cigarettes to remove branding from cigarette packets. Called 'plain packaging' in fact branding has been replaced by disturbing graphic images showing the insides of smokers' lungs. At the time of this proposal, it was admitted that there was limited evidence as to whether it would dissuade people from smoking and especially whether it would stop young people from starting to smoke (Chantler 2014). So far the evidence of the effectiveness of this intervention in stopping people from smoking remains weak (Lilic, Stretton and Prakash 2018; McNeill et al. 2017; Underwood, Sun and Welters 2020). However, studies have shown that the packaging raised awareness of the dangers of smoking amongst young non-smokers (Drovandi et al. 2019) and made the pack less appealing to all (Gravely et al. 2021), but it seems that the price of cigarettes remains the most effective disincentive to smoking (Doogan, Wewers and Berman 2017; Yeh et al. 2017).

The Ethics of Fear Appeal

Plain cigarette packaging is an example of negative campaigning. This presentation of dire warnings to people is termed fear appeal, that failure to act on a health message will result in bad consequences for the individual. The problem with using tactics which generate disgust such as the plain packaging rule is that a link is made between disgust and the individual. People who are overweight can be fat shamed, for example, feeling the disgust of other people and maybe feeling disgust about themselves due to the narrative which is being adopted by others (Lupton 2015). Such feelings are more likely to ostracise people from society and stop them seeking help which is counterproductive, and hence these tactics are bordering on the unethical due to their negative impact (Peters, Ruiter and Kok 2014). Advertising for public health especially in mass media campaigns can be a blunt instrument. Old ladies who don't drive tune in to television adverts and see distressing pictures of children being injured in road traffic accidents caused by speeding drivers, and life-long non-smokers see smokers gasping for breath. Complaints made to the advertising standards authority have resulted in some adverts being withdrawn. In 2007, a UK anti-smoking advert which showed people with fish hooks through their lips attracted the largest number of complaints from the public (774) that year and was consequently withdrawn. The advertisement which implied that smokers were hooked on cigarettes was shown to have been offensive, frightening and distressing (The Guardian 2007). It is important to consider how people respond to health messages. Research has shown that exposure to negative health messages can cause stress. The ability to cope with this exposure varies from individual to individual, but those from lower socio-economic groups are more likely than those from higher socio-economic groups to respond by either blocking out the message or accepting the message, but then feeling that they do not have the ability or resources to act on the message (Iversen and Kraft 2006). It is also important to be truthful when presenting health messages and avoid both sensationalism and censure. Sweeping statements such as 'smoking cannabis will give you schizophrenia' belies people's experience of taking the drug or the knowledge of others who have taken it safely. This leads to public mistrust of the agencies who are presenting this message and credibility once lost is hard to regain.

Positive Messaging

O'Keefe and Jensen (2008) performed a systematic review looking at gain framed (positive benefits gained by adopting certain healthy behaviours) versus loss framed (negative consequences resulting from unhealthy behaviours) message presentation. They failed to prove that loss framed messages were any more engaging than gained framed messages. People appeared to be more engaged when the benefits of positive actions for health were presented to them rather than when the key aspect of the message focused on negative consequences of certain actions or inactions. This was especially noticeable when the message focused on the prevention of disease. Gradually social marketers are moving away from such fear tactics and are presenting positive messages emphasising the benefits of changing instead. Stoptober is a UK promotional campaign to encourage smokers to stop for the month of October. The campaign is based on the research that people who quit for a 28-day period have a high success rate of remaining non-smokers. Stoptober utilises the positive effects of a mass movement and increased social support, and it uses digital prompts and achievable personal goal setting apps to increase and sustain motivation. Research has shown that this positive approach works in that it greatly increases quit attempts during the month of October. In 2018, this was 19% of all English smokers; however, the number who were still stopped at four weeks was only 8% (Public Health England 2019). This emphasises the point that campaigns can only raise awareness and increase motivation, and longer term help is needed to support people through the ups and downs of behaviour change. The question remains as to why governments, health departments and organisations persist in presenting fear appeal messages when there is little evidence that these result in significant behaviour change. Is it because society seems to have more of a natural predilection for punishment than reward? If so, it is a sad indictment, but one look at health policy leaves the reader in no doubt that this is the case. There are many examples of health legislation to force compliance with healthy behaviours, for example, speed limits, seat belt laws, not smoking in public places and taxation to punish the unhealthy behaviours of drinking alcohol and smoking. Less in evidence are incentives to reward people for indulging in healthy behaviours. In fact, these, such as eating a healthy diet and undertaking regular physical activity, have costs associated with them.

   The debate regarding persuasive messages is not a new one. In 1908, two psychologists, Yerkes and Dodson, studied optimal levels of arousal that were associated with optimal levels of performance or behaviour change. Experiments were conducted which subjected people in a study to various stimuli, some of which were at a low level and others were more challenging, thereby resulting in higher levels of arousal in these individuals. They found that people responded best and were most likely to act on messages which were interesting, but not off-putting. If the way that the message was packaged was boring, people didn't remember it; however, if it was too shocking, people blocked it out. There, therefore, seems to be an ideal level of arousal somewhere in the middle which grabs people's interest without upsetting them, and it was this middle level of stimulation which equated with the most instances of behaviour change. Researchers are still testing out the Yerkes-Dodson law in respect to the level of stimulus compared with behaviour change and finding the relationship is still proven (Johnson et al. 2012).

Edutainment

Samuel Goldwyn, a famous Hollywood film producer in the 1930s and 1940s, once declared that 'films are for entertainment, messages should be delivered by Western Union' (BBC 2013). Nevertheless, the media industry has the potential to be an important ally in health promotion, and the combination of education and entertainment has given rise to the term edutainment as when an entertainment programme also seeks to deliver a message to its audience. Examples of this are storylines in soap operas. Obviously, this has to be subtlety done and the storylines need to be credible and entertaining. Research into effectiveness of integrating health messages into soap operas has shown that the audience connects to characters whose lives they follow and that messages that are relatable are retained for long periods (Bhebhe 2022). It is important of course that such stories have a good factual underpinning so as not to mislead audiences for the sake of dramatic content or reinforce stereotypes. Professionals knowledgeable about the issues involved should be consulted regarding scripts and audience reactions sought. Public health departments around the world are realising that in order to get audience attention, messages need to be entertaining, amusing and have high quality creative content just like the entertainment industry. During the COVID-19 pandemic, US Public Health Departments produced a series of animations reinforcing the need for social distancing and showing viral spread, which were proved to be engaging, humorous and effective (Adam and Gates 2020). Boring, expert led messages will not engage people and not get results.

Use of Digital Technology and Social Media

Wearable Devices

In recent times, the growth of digital technology has also seen a growth in gadgets to promote health and well-being. Wearable devices which monitor diet, physical activity and sleep patterns have become increasingly popular. Research is showing that these can have a positive impact on increasing physical activity levels, at least in the short term (Larsen et al. 2022; Singh, Zopf and Howden 2022; Tang et al. 2020). However, the usefulness and accuracy of the calorie expenditure functions seem to vary widely between manufacturers and also the type of exercise undertaken and are generally acknowledged to still be inaccurate (Maher et al. 2017; Shcherbina et al. 2017; Woodland 2021). The sleep monitoring function is also problematic as the devices are usually worn on the wrist and monitor movement which is not always an accurate way of monitoring sleep patterns. There is also disturbing research to show that routinely being told that your sleep is poor by these devices can result in feelings of low mood and anxiety, whether or not these devices are accurate or not (Gavriloff et al. 2018; Reid 2021). There is also the probability that the consumers of wearable devices are already motivated towards health and fitness, so although they may be a good tool for monitoring physical activity, they will hardly appeal to sedentary individuals.

Health Applications

Health apps such as mHealth applications on smartphones are booming and include apps on a whole range of physical and mental health issues. Again, these need to be proactively sought out by users. Research has shown that those which allow users to set their own goals, have clear instructions and are easy to navigate and simple to use have the best customer experience and are most likely to result in longer periods of use (Vaghefi and Tulu 2019). In the UK, the NHS Food scanner app can be used in supermarkets to suggest healthier food alternatives, and there is also an NHS weight loss plan app and many mental health apps (Alqahtani et al. 2019; NHS Choices 2022a). The weight reduction apps have shown some success in the short term (Ghelani et al. 2020; Innes et al. 2019), although sustainability of weight loss is always an issue. Client motivation remains the key factor in the success of these apps and the standard and cost to the public varied considerably (Fitzgerald and Mc-Clelland 2017). At present, the research citing the effectiveness of such apps is inconclusive (Milne-Ives et al., 2020; O'Neil 2019; Wisniewski et al., 2019), but at the very least the popularity of these applications show that many people are proactively seeking out ways to improve their health.

Social Media

Social media such as social network sites and health forums, blogs and message boards are seen as having an increasing role in the dissemination and discussion of health promotion issues (Jane et al. 2018). Social media such as Twitter or online health forums can gather data from its community regarding knowledge and opinions of health concerns and test out thoughts regarding possible interventions. Specific Facebook pages for people with a common health issue or interest in common, for example, parents of autistic children, can be used to disseminate information and social media can be used to galvanise support, raise awareness and funding for certain issues, fun runs for breast cancer research for instance. At present, much of the health promotion content using social media platforms tends to be purely informative and users have requested more interactive content (O'Neil 2019; Richards, Woodcox and Forster 2022). Websites seem to be more interactive, but require users to search for such sites (NHS Choices 2022b), whereas using platforms that people are already a member of means that messages are delivered automatically. Receipt of such content may result in a negative annoyance value, but users are so used to sponsored advertisements that so as long as the content is respectful and not shocking hopefully any irritation can be minimised. This mass marketing however comes at a cost and the effectiveness of using social media in health promotion is yet to be fully explored.

Activity

Watch a health information advert, either on TV, the internet or on social media.

- Is the message positively or negatively portrayed?
- Who do you think the message is aimed at?

- Would the message be inappropriate or even upsetting if viewed by a vulnerable person, e.g. a child? An adult with learning disabilities? Someone with a mental health diagnosis?
- Does the advert provide information?
- Does the advert point the viewer in the direction of services to help them should they decide to act on the message?
- Do you think it raises awareness of the issue?
- Do you think that the message is clear?
- Did the message engage with you or make you switch off?
- Do you think the advert was ethical?

Critical Thinking

As we know more about what causes ill health, are we less tolerant of unhealthy lifestyles than we used to be?

As we have seen so far, knowledge of health determinants doesn't automatically lead to changes to the adoption of healthier behaviours and many people do not possess the ability to change. Is it therefore ethical to constantly bombard people with health information when they are not in a position to act?

Are health promoters merely adding to social injustice by dumping the problem at individuals' doorsteps, especially when society allows smoking, drinking and overeating yet censures those who do this?

The alternative is to restrict information, thereby denying those motivated and capable of change from help in doing so. What is needed from health promoters is an intelligent reading of the whole picture and not a simplistic victim blaming approach. Rather than despairing at people's apparent weakness or lack of self-responsibility, health promoters need to develop the capacity, skills and effective techniques to work with individuals seeking to change whilst lobbying for national and local policies to make these changes easier to make.

Key Messages

- A wide variety of mechanisms exist for disseminating health information.
- We are all potential health educators, virtually everyone can informally impart health messages, but for the wider health and social care workforce, it forms an essential part of their role.
- Mass media, digital technology and social media all have the potential to disseminate and debate health issues, but users need to be able to assess the quality of information provided.
- Increased knowledge as to health determinants may lead to victim blaming which is both unhelpful and unethical.
- Health educators need to possess sound knowledge, update this and be able to signpost people onto appropriate services and sources of information.

References

Adam, M. and Gates, J. (2020). *The rise of 'health entertainment' to convey lifesaving messages in the COVID-19 pandemic* [online]. Scientific American Blog Network. Available at: https://blogs.scientificamerican.com/observations/the-rise-of-health-entertainment-to-convey-lifesaving-messages-in-the-covid-19-pandemic/

Alqahtani, F., Al Khalifah, G., Oyebode, O. and Orji, R. (2019). Apps for mental health: An evaluation of behavior change strategies and recommendations for future development. *Frontiers in Artificial Intelligence* [online], 2. Available at: https://www.frontiersin.org/articles/10.3389/frai.2019.00030/full

Battineni, G., Baldoni, S., Chintalapudi, N., Sagaro, G.G., Pallotta, G., Nittari, G. and Amenta, F. (2020). Factors affecting the quality and reliability of online health information. *Digital Health* [online], 6, p. 205520762094899. Available at: https://journals.sagepub.com/doi/full/10.1177/2055207620948996 [accessed 14 March 2022].

BBC. (2013). BBC radio 4, *The film programme* 18th April. London. BBC.

Becker, H. (1999). Informed decision making: An annotated bibliography and systematic review. *Health technology assessment*; Vol. 3: No.1

Benware, C. (1984). Quality of learning with an active versus passive motivational set. *American Educational Research Journal*, 21(4), pp. 755–765.

Bhebhe, A. (2022). Soap operas can deliver effective health education to young people – new research [online]. *The Conversation*. Available at: https://theconversation.com/soap-operas-can-deliver-effective-health-education-to-young-people-new-research-175087

Chantler, C. (2014). *Standardised packaging of tobacco report of the independent review undertaken by Sir Cyril Chantler* [online]. Available at: https://www.kcl.ac.uk/health/10035-TSO-2901853-Chantler-Review-ACCESSIBLE.PDF

Cheng, H., Kotler, P. and Lee, N.R. (2009) *Social marketing for health: An introduction.* Burlington MA. Jones and Bartlett.

David, S. and Pinch, T. (2006). Six degrees of reputation: The use and abuse of online review and recommendation systems. *First Monday*, 11(3). https://doi.org/10.5210/fm.v11i3.1315

Doogan, N.J., Wewers, M.E. and Berman, M. (2017). The impact of a federal cigarette minimum pack price policy on cigarette use in the USA. *Tobacco Control* [online], 27(2), pp. 203–208. Available at: https://pubmed.ncbi.nlm.nih.gov/28259846/

Drovandi, A., Teague, P.-A., Glass, B. and Malau-Aduli, B. (2019). A systematic review of the perceptions of adolescents on graphic health warnings and plain packaging of cigarettes. *Systematic Reviews* [online], 8(1). Available at: https://systematicreviewsjournal.biomedcentral.com/articles/10.1186/s13643-018-0933-0

Firestone, R., Rowe, C., Modi, S. and Sievers, D. (2017). The effectiveness of social marketing in global health: A systematic review. *Health Policy and Planning*, 32 (1), 110–124, https://doi.org/10.1093/heapol/czw088

Fitzgerald, M. and McClelland, T. (2017). What makes a mobile app successful in supporting health behaviour change? *Health Education Journal*, 76(3), pp. 373–381.

Gavriloff, D., Sheaves, B., Juss, A., Espie, C.A., Miller, C.B. and Kyle, S.D. (2018). Sham sleep feedback delivered via actigraphy biases daytime symptom reports in people with insomnia: Implications for insomnia disorder and wearable devices. *Journal of Sleep Research* [online], 27(6), p. e12726. Available at: https://pubmed.ncbi.nlm.nih.gov/29989248/

Ghelani, D.P., Moran, L.J., Johnson, C., Mousa, A. and Naderpoor, N. (2020). Mobile Apps for weight management: A review of the latest evidence to inform practice. *Frontiers in Endocrinology* [online], 11. Available at: https://www.ncbi.nlm.nih.gov/pmc/articles/PMC7326765/#:~:text=Results%20showed%20a%20positive%20change,and%20change%20in%20energy%20intake

GOV.UK. (2021). *Promotions of unhealthy foods restricted from October 2022* [online]. GOV.UK. Available at: https://www.gov.uk/government/news/promotions-of-unhealthy-foods-restricted-from-october-2022

Gravely, S., Chung-Hall, J., Craig, L.V., Fong, G.T., Cummings, K.M., Borland, R., Yong, H.-H., Loewen, R., Martin, N., Quah, A.C.K., Hammond, D., Ouimet, J., Boudreau, C., Thompson, M.E.

and Driezen, P. (2021). Evaluating the impact of plain packaging among Canadian smokers: Findings from the 2018 and 2020 ITC smoking and vaping surveys. *Tobacco Control* [online], tobaccocontrol-2021-056635. Available at: https://tobaccocontrol.bmj.com/content/early/2021/10/19/tobaccocontrol-2021-056635

Griebel, L., Enwald, H., Gilstad, H., Pohl, A.-L., Moreland, J. and Sedlmayr, M. (2017). eHealth literacy research—Quo vadis? *Informatics for Health and Social Care* [online], 43(4), pp. 427–442. Available at: https://pubmed.ncbi.nlm.nih.gov/29045164/

Hu, N., Liu, L. Jr., Sambamurthy, V. and Chen, B. (2009). *Are online reviews just noise? The truth, the whole truth, or only the partial truth*. Singapore Management University. https://ink.library.smu.edu.sg/sis_research/338/.

Huxley, A. (1932) *Brave new world*. London: Chatto and Windus.

Innes, A.Q., Thomson, G., Cotter, M., King, J.A., Vollaard, N.B.J. and Kelly, B.M. (2019). Evaluating differences in the clinical impact of a free online weight loss programme, a resource-intensive commercial weight loss programme and an active control condition: A parallel randomised controlled trial. *BMC Public Health* [online], 19(1). Available at: https://bmcpublichealth.biomedcentral.com/articles/10.1186/s12889-019-8061-x

Iversen, C.A. and Kraft, P. (2006). Does socio-economic status and health consciousness influence how women respond to health related messages in media? *Health Education Research*, 21(5), pp. 601–610.

Jane, M., Hagger, M., Foster, J., Ho, S. and Pal, S. (2018). Social media for health promotion and weight management: A critical debate. *BMC Public Health* [online], 18(1). Available at: https://bmcpublichealth.biomedcentral.com/articles/10.1186/s12889-018-5837-3

Johnson, C., Moreno, J., Regas, K., Tyler, C. and Foreyt, J. (2012). The application of the Yerkes–Dodson law in a childhood weight management program: Examining weight dissatisfaction. *Journal of Paediatric Psychology*, 37(6), pp. 674–679.

Jungmin, P. and Zuniga, J. (2016). Effectiveness of using picture-based health education for people with low health literacy: An integrative review. *Cogent Medicine* [online]. Available at: https://www.tandfonline.com/doi/full/10.1080/2331205X.2016.1264679

Keçeci, A., Toprak, S. and Kiliç, S. (2017). How effective are patient education materials in educating patients? *Clinical Nursing Research* [online], 28(5), pp. 567–582. Available at: https://journals.sagepub.com/doi/abs/10.1177/1054773817740521

Kerr, J., Eves, F. and Carroll, D. (2000). Posters can prompt less active people to use the stairs. *Journal of Epidemiological and Community Health*, 54, pp. 942–943.

Kolb, D.A. (1984). *Experiential learning: Experience as the source of learning and development*. Englewood Cliffs, NJ: Prentice Hall.

Kotler, P. and Lee, N.R. (2008). *Social marketing: Influencing behaviours for good*. 3rd ed. Thousand Oaks, CA: Sage.

Kuipers, M.A.G., Beard, E., West, R. and Brown, J. (2017). Associations between tobacco control mass media campaign expenditure and smoking prevalence and quitting in England: A time series analysis. *Tobacco Control* [online], 27(4), pp. 455–462. Available at: https://pubmed.ncbi.nlm.nih.gov/28667091/

Larsen, R.T., Wagner, V., Korfitsen, C.B., Keller, C., Juhl, C.B., Langberg, H. and Christensen, J. (2022). Effectiveness of physical activity monitors in adults: Systematic review and meta-analysis. *BMJ* [online], p. e068047. Available at: https://www.bmj.com/content/376/bmj-2021-068047

Leiner, M., Handel, G. and Williams, D. (2004). Patient communication: A multidisciplinary approach using animated cartoons. *Health Education Research*, 19(5), pp. 591–595.

Lilic, N., Stretton, M. and Prakash, M. (2018). How effective is the plain packaging of tobacco policy on rates of intention to quit smoking and changing attitudes to smoking? *ANZ Journal of Surgery* [online], 88(9), pp. 825–830. Available at: https://pubmed.ncbi.nlm.nih.gov/29873162/

Lupton, D. (2015). The pedagogy of disgust: The ethical, moral and political implications of using disgust in public health campaigns. *Critical Public Health* [online]. Available at: https://www.tandfonline.com/doi/abs/10.1080/09581596.2014.885115

Maher, C., Ryan, J., Ambrosi, C. and Edney, S. (2017). Users' experiences of wearable activity trackers: A cross-sectional study. *BMC Public Health* [online], 17(1). Available at: https://bmcpub lichealth.biomedcentral.com/articles/10.1186/s12889-017-4888-1

Maskell, K., McDonald, P. and Paudyal, P. (2018). Effectiveness of health education materials in general practice waiting rooms: A cross-sectional study. *British Journal of General Practice* [online], 68(677), pp. e869–e876. Available at: https://bjgp.org/content/early/2018/10/22/bjgp18X699773/tab-pdf?versioned=true

McNeill, A., Gravely, S., Hitchman, S.C., Bauld, L., Hammond, D. and Hartmann-Boyce, J. (2017). Tobacco packaging design for reducing tobacco use. *Cochrane Database of Systematic Reviews* [online], 2017(4). Available at: https://www.cochranelibrary.com/cdsr/doi/10.1002/14651858. CD011244.pub2/full

Meade, C.D., McKinney, W.P. and Barnas, G.P. (1994). Educating patients with limited literacy skills: The effectiveness of printed and videotaped materials about colon cancer. *American Journal of Public Health*, 84(1), pp. 119–121.

Milne-Ives, M., Lam, C., De Cock, C., Van Velthoven, M.H. and Meinert, E. (2020). Mobile apps for health behavior change in physical activity, diet, drug and alcohol use, and mental health: Systematic review. *JMIR mHealth and uHealth* [online], 8(3), p. e17046. Available at: https://mhealth. jmir.org/2020/3/e17046/

MRC Epidemiology Unit. (2021). *Sugar purchased in soft drinks fell 10% following introduction of industry levy - MRC Epidemiology Unit* [online]. Available at: https://www.mrc-epid.cam.ac.uk/blog/2021/03/11/sugar-purchased-in-soft-drinks-fell-10-following-introduction-of-industry-levy/

National Institute Health and Care Research (NIHR) Evidence. (2019). *Mixed evidence shows some impact of mass media campaigns promoting tobacco control, physical activity and sexual health - NIHR Evidence* [online]. Available at: https://evidence.nihr.ac.uk/alert/mixed-evidence-shows-some-impact-of-mass-media-campaigns-promoting-tobacco-control-physical-activity-and-sexual-health/

Nccmt.ca. (2013). *Assessing health communication messages | NCCMT.* [online] Available at: https://www.nccmt.ca/knowledge-repositories/search/63

NHS Choices. (2022a). *Lose weight* [online]. Available at: https://www.nhs.uk/better-health/lose-weight/?WT.mc_ID=SEARCH_LOSEWEIGHT&gclid=EAIaIQobChMIl-Hdod_F9gIVj-7t Ch3nQgoDEAAYASAAEgI-n_D_BwE&gclsrc=aw.ds

NHS Choices. (2022b). *Better health – Healthier families home* [online]. Available at: https://www. nhs.uk/healthier-families/

O'Keefe, D.J. and Jensen, J.D. (2008). Do loss-framed persuasive messages engender greater message processing than do gain-framed messages? A meta-analytic review. *Communication Studies*, 59(1), pp. 51–61.

O'Neil, I. (2019). *Digital health promotion.* Cambridge. Polity.

Peters, G.Y., Ruiter, R.A.C. and Kok, G. (2014). Threatening communication: A qualitative study of fear appeal effectiveness beliefs among intervention developers, policymakers, politicians, scientists, and advertising professionals. *International Journal of Psychology* [online], 49(2), pp. 71–79. Available at: https://www.ncbi.nlm.nih.gov/pmc/articles/PMC4278564/

Public Health England. (2019). *Stoptober 2018: Campaign evaluation.* https://assets.publishing. service.gov.uk/government/uploads/system/uploads/attachment_data/file/835518/Stoptober_2018_ evaluation.pdf

Reid, M. (2021). Are sleep trackers accurate? Here's what researchers currently know [online]. *The Conversation.* Available at: https://theconversation.com/are-sleep-trackers-accurate-heres-what-researchers-currently-know-152500#:~:text=Despite%20their%20popularity%2C%20only%20 a,when%20identifying%20sleep%20versus%20wakefulness

Richards, E.A., Woodcox, S. and Forster, A. (2022). What works and for whom? Outcome evaluation of an e-mail walking program delivered through cooperative extension. *Journal of Primary Care & Community Health* [online], 13, p. 215013192110706. Available at: https://pubmed.ncbi.nlm.nih. gov/35094592/

Rudd, R.E. and Comings, J.P. (1994). Learner developed materials: An empowering approach. *Health Education Quarterly*, 21(3), pp. 313–327.

Shcherbina, A., Mattsson, C., Waggott, D., Salisbury, H., Christle, J., Hastie, T., Wheeler, M. and Ashley, E. (2017). Accuracy in wrist-worn, sensor-based measurements of heart rate and energy expenditure in a diverse cohort. *Journal of Personalized Medicine* [online], 7(2), p. 3. Available at: https://www.mdpi.com/2075-4426/7/2/3

Sims, M., Salway, R., Langley, T., Lewis, S., McNeill, A., Szatkowski, L. and Gilmore, A.B. (2014). Effectiveness of tobacco control television advertising in changing tobacco use in England: A population-based cross-sectional study. *Addiction* [online], 109(6), pp. 986–994. Available at: https://pubmed.ncbi.nlm.nih.gov/24467285/

Singh, B., Zopf, E.M. and Howden, E.J. (2022). Effect and feasibility of wearable physical activity trackers and pedometers for increasing physical activity and improving health outcomes in cancer survivors: A systematic review and meta-analysis. *Journal of Sport and Health Science* [online], 11(2), pp. 184–193. Available at: https://www.sciencedirect.com/science/article/pii/S2095254621 000909#:~:text=Preliminary%20evidence%20suggests%20that%20wearable,tools%20that%20 increase%20activity%20levels.&text=These%20devices%20provide%20feedback%20on, and%20record%20and%20review%20data

Somadi F. (2023). Sports business sponsorship. We live and breath chocolate and football. Available at: https://sponsorship.sportbusiness.com/2023/04/we-live-and-breathe-chocolate-and-football-nicholas-rogers-cadbury/

Sport Business Sponsorship. (2022). Organisation: Cadbury | SportBusiness Sponsorship [online]. *SportBusiness Sponsorship*. Available at: https://sponsorship.sportbusiness.com/organisation/cadbury/

Tang, M.S.S., Moore, K., McGavigan, A., Clark, R.A. and Ganesan, A.N. (2020). Effectiveness of wearable trackers on physical activity in healthy adults: Systematic review and meta-analysis of randomized controlled trials. *JMIR mHealth and uHealth* [online], 8(7), p. e15576. Available at: https://www.ncbi.nlm.nih.gov/pmc/articles/PMC7407266/

The Guardian. (2007). Anti-smoking *ads hooked off air* [online]. The Guardian. Available at: https://www.theguardian.com/media/2007/may/16/advertising.uknews.

Underwood, D., Sun, S. and Welters, R.A.M.H.M. (2020). The effectiveness of plain packaging in discouraging tobacco consumption in Australia. *Nature Human Behaviour* [online], 4(12), pp. 1273–1284. Available at: https://www.nature.com/articles/s41562-020-00940-6

Vaghefi, I. and Tulu, B. (2019). The continued use of Mobile health apps: Insights from a longitudinal study. *JMIR mHealth and uHealth* [online], 7(8), p. e12983. Available at: https://www.ncbi.nlm.nih.gov/pmc/articles/PMC6740166/

Ward, K. and Hawthorne, K. (1994). Do patients read health promotion posters in the waiting room? A study in one general practice. *British Journal of General Practice*, 44(389), pp. 583–585.

WHO. (2019). *European roadmap for implementation of health literacy initiatives through the life course*. 69th session of the WHO Regional Committee for Europe, 16–19 September 2019.

Wicke, D.M., Lorge, R.E., Coppin, R.J. and Jones, K.P. (1994). The effectiveness of waiting room notice-boards as a vehicle for health education. *Family Practitioner*, 11, pp. 292–295.

Wisniewski, H., Liu, G., Henson, P., Vaidyam, A., Hajratalli, N.K., Onnela, J.-P. and Torous, J. (2019). Understanding the quality, effectiveness and attributes of top-rated smartphone health apps. *Evidence Based Mental Health* [online], 22(1), pp. 4–9. Available at: https://ebmh.bmj.com/content/22/1/4

Woodland, R. (2021). *How accurate are fitness trackers?* [online]. livescience.com. Available at: https://www.livescience.com/how-accurate-are-fitness-trackers

Yeh, C.-Y., Schafferer, C., Lee, J.-M., Ho, L.-M. and Hsieh, C.-J. (2017). The effects of a rise in cigarette price on cigarette consumption, tobacco taxation revenues, and of smoking-related deaths in 28 EU countries– applying threshold regression modelling. *BMC Public Health* [online], 17(1). Available at: https://bmcpublichealth.biomedcentral.com/articles/10.1186/s12889-017-4685-x

7 Supporting People Through Behaviour Change

Susan R. Thompson and Mo Lockwood

Introduction

Five key lifestyle factors combined – never having smoked, not being overweight, undertaking regular physical activity, not drinking excessive alcohol and having a good quality diet – have been shown to increase healthy life expectancy by 10 years in women and 7.6 years in men (Bmj.com 2020). Individuals concentrating on these specific health behaviours, therefore, have a lot to gain. Working directly with clients to help them achieve behaviour change is an important part of health promotion and public health work. Whether it be nurses working with their patients, or health workers with a specialist remit in certain areas such as smoking cessation or drug and alcohol misuse, supporting individuals through behaviour change forms an essential part of health promotion practice. To help workers support their clients and patients successfully, a range of techniques and tools have been developed. The important starting point when commencing work with people on behaviour change is to assess the client's level of knowledge regarding health determinants and also their level of motivation for change. Motivation arises either from intrinsic (from ourselves, driven by our wants and sense of satisfaction and enjoyment) or extrinsic (suggested to us by others to avoid punishment or get rewards) sources (Swanson and Maltinsky 2019). Both aspects of motivation work together, but it is important that health promoters generate enjoyment and a sense of satisfaction (intrinsic) as well as advising (extrinsic) which can put individuals under too much pressure (Simply Psychology.org). It is essential to act as a facilitator. The health promoter should support their client to set their own agenda and goals and should not dictate to clients. This is not only unethical, but also it doesn't work as people cannot be made to change unless they want to.

For people to consider behaviour change, they need to connect to a health message and see it as relevant to themselves. Sometimes the message only gets through when life circumstances change and the person concerned is able to connect it and see its implications for their own life. Life events can act as a catalyst for behaviour change (Bhattacharya et al. 2018). This could be a change in someone's personal health, a health scare which could contradict the 'it couldn't happen to me' mentality that we often subconsciously believe. Possibly, a non-cancerous breast lump may cause a woman to cut down on her alcohol intake and regularly check her breasts for any changes. Other personal issues may be a realisation of our own deteriorating health, possibly a long-term smoker now notices that he gets out of breath very quickly and therefore decides to quit. Other situations that may spur people on to consider behaviour change may be the change in the health of a friend or family member. The presence of a serious health condition so close to home may serve as a wake-up call, especially if that person is of the same age and gender. Another circumstance that may cause people to consider behaviour change may be assuming responsibility for someone

DOI: 10.4324/9781003411321-7

else, prospective new parents may consider stopping smoking and a pregnant woman may decide not to drink alcohol and to eat more healthily.

The Health Belief Model

Research has shown that when people are considering change, they weigh up the costs and benefits to themselves of making the change. This is the premise of the Health Belief Model (Nutbeam and Harris 2004). This model suggests that, first of all, people estimate their susceptibility to a particular health issue. If they are indulging in risk-taking behaviour, they consider the likelihood of this behaviour causing that health issue for them. This is heavily influenced by an individual's attitude. For example, they may feel that they can still drive fast and won't be involved in an accident, so they will continue to drive fast as they don't perceive themselves as susceptible. Young people may smoke because they don't perceive heart disease as a threat, at least for them, they can always quit later. Next, people consider the seriousness of the possible problem, that is, 'if I get this health problem how life limiting will this be?' 'what would this mean for me?' Again, they may decide that the risk is acceptable and continue. After this, people weigh up what they may gain by changing their behaviour compared with what they may lose. It may seem obvious that people will gain more than they would lose by adopting healthy behaviours but this may not be the case, especially in the short term. It's all to do with the matter of perception. Someone who quits smoking may even in the short term feel fitter, but they will lose their smoking break at work with their mates. It is often this change in social networks which can make people think twice about instigating change. A person who drinks too much alcohol may have to change his social circle, for example. Thus, people tend to weigh up the perceived benefits, threats and anticipated outcomes of change before they embark on any change. Importantly though before people enter into change, they need to feel that it is within their power to actually change their behaviour. They need to believe that they possess the willpower, strategies, resources and support to be successful. This confidence in the ability to succeed is termed self-efficacy. If people don't believe this, they won't even attempt change (Schunk and DiBenedetto 2021). Our job as health promoters is to help people with this decision-making process, increase self-efficacy and facilitate empowerment by providing support and practical help for change. Figure 7.1 shows how an individual may follow the health belief model when weighing up the pros and cons of adopting safe sexual practices in an attempt to lessen his or her risk of becoming HIV positive.

Behaviour Change Frameworks

There are a variety of tools or frameworks to aid health promoters in helping people with behaviour change. There is much similarity between these different frameworks and generally they all have at their core the key recommended principles of goal setting, planning, feedback, monitoring and social support (National Institute for Health and Care Excellence (NICE) 2020). Individuals need to be assessed regarding their needs and preferences and their capability, opportunity and motivation for change. This is often referred to as the COM B model (National Institute for Health and Care Excellence (NICE) 2020). Given below is a discussion of some techniques in common use.

Brief Advice

Another important catalyst for people starting to undertake behaviour change and one which is important for health professionals to be aware of is that the public respond to being advised to change their behaviour by someone who is respected and seen as knowledgeable.

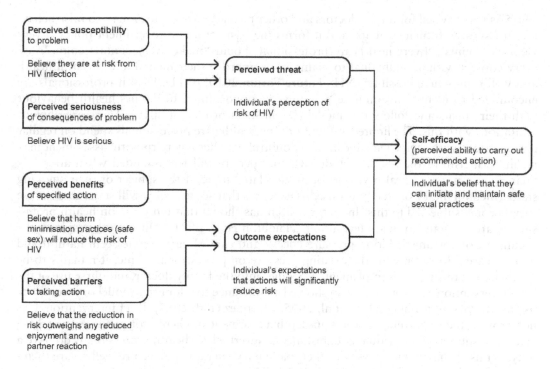

Figure 7.1 Adaptation of The Health Belief Model (Rosenstock, Strecher and Becker 1988) with Regard to HIV

A systematic review of research studies has shown that brief advice from a health professional lasting no more than three minutes has been shown to increase a person's chance of quitting smoking by up to 3% (Cochrane Collaboration 2008). This may be seen as a relatively small percentage, but taken on a population level and considering the number of people in day-to-day contact with health professionals, it equates to a large number of people for such a quick and easy intervention. Obviously, this percentage can be increased by signposting people to specialist services and providing longer, more in-depth consultations. One example of this brief advice or invention technique is the 5As model (ask, advise, assess, assist and arrange). The model encourages health care workers to the following:

Ask: Raise an issue with their clients, for example, 'Do you smoke?'

Advise: Provide information regarding the hazards of smoking and advise quitting.

Assess: Assess the client's motivation to change. This could be done by questioning, for example, 'On a scale of 1-10 how motivated are you to quit at the moment?' This stage should also include the assessment of the client's pattern of smoking, their previous quit attempts, etc.

Assist: This is the action planning stage in which the health promoter and the client work together to set goals and agree on a strategy to achieve these goals. This will include information on the support services and resources available to aid the client in their behaviour change. Client confidence with this action plan may be assessed by asking the question, 'On a scale of 1-10 how confident are you of being able to quit?'

Arrange: This stage involves referral or signposting to specialist services, for example, a specialist smoking cessation service.

The 5As was devised for use by doctors and other primary care professionals to raise behavioural issues with their patients, and it forms the basis of a UK government policy 'Every Contact Counts', 'Every healthcare professional should "make every contact count": use every contact with an individual to maintain or improve their mental and physical health and wellbeing where possible' (NHS Future Forum 2010, p. 11). Health professionals are encouraged to identify five-minute 'windows of opportunity' to discuss health behaviour with their clients and follow this model (Department of Health 2010). There are obvious limitations with this. The limited amount of time health care professionals spend on regular consultations with their clients means it is doubtful whether any purposeful assessment may result. Criticism of the policy includes whether people will feel hounded when attending their doctor, nurse or health visitor for an unrelated topic, if the subject of their smoking status, alcohol intake or weight is raised. The fear is that some people will stay away in case they become subjected to this. In fact, research has shown that ten years on health professionals are resistant to this intervention (Haighton et al. 2021). On the other side of the argument, opportunistic blood pressure checks and chat about lifestyle seem natural and holistic care. However, with the existing pressure on professionals' time, it remains to be seen whether this policy is implemented. Studies into the family doctor and nurse use of the brief intervention 5As approach also showed a reluctance to adopt this model or incomplete use due to lack of training (Dosh et al. 2005; Martínez et al. 2017). Brief intervention does not provide the opportunity for any in-depth assessment of client motivation or matching goals and support to individual circumstances. Nevertheless, health professionals do have a duty to raise behavioural issues with their patients. Generally, people are well aware themselves of the basic healthy messages. So this brief intervention is perhaps best used in signposting people to more specialist health promotion services which can spend more time with patients and provide them with an in-depth assessment of their own individual needs and provide the necessary continuing support for behaviour change.

Critical Thinking

Take some time out to think about and research the following:

Does providing statins and other preventative medicine just give people a licence to act irresponsibly?

Is this fair that those who follow behaviour change advice have to pay via their taxes for treatment for those who don't?

The Transtheoretical Model (Stages of Change)

For more in-depth work with clients on behaviour change, Prochaska and Di Clemente's model is a well-recognised and commonly used behavioural change tool (Prochaska and Di-Clemente 1984). The model begins by assessing the client's motivation to change, and questions are asked of the client, such as 'Have you ever thought that you perhaps needed to cut down your alcohol intake? Or, 'Do you feel like you would like to lose some weight?' It is important that such questions are raised without making a judgement and in a chatty open manner. The client's reply to exploratory questions allows the health promoter to categorise the client as being in a particular stage of the cycle of change. They may answer that they do not want to change, in which case Prochaska and DiClemente would categorise them as being in the pre-contemplation stage, not interested in changing at the present time. If this is the case, the health promoter's best response would be along the lines of 'Well if you do ever get to the stage when you are considering changing, please come and see me because there is a lot of help we can give you to help you quit smoking'. They might reply that they would like to quit but doubt that they would be successful, or have tried before and failed. They would then be categorised as being in the contemplation phase of the cycle. It is the health promoter's job in this case to build up their confidence, undertake a detailed assessment of their circumstances and habits and work with them to move them to the next stage of the cycle, the planning stage. In this stage, any previous history of change attempts is explored, what helped? what do they think went wrong? etc., and goals are set and action plans drawn up. With smoking cessation, this will involve setting a quit date and deciding on the use of pharmaceutical products, such as nicotine replacement therapy, bupropion or vareni-cline to help with nicotine withdrawal symptoms. The next stage, making changes, is to put the plan into action with the ongoing support of the health promoter. This means regular follow-up appointments and a reassessment of the action plan with changes made as neces-sary. Hopefully, the client will then enter the maintenance phase and adopt the long-term behaviour change, again with the help of follow-up appointments as necessary. Successful long-term behaviour changes lasting for six months or more will then mean that they will exit the cycle. However, many people relapse and go into this stage of the cycle. Relapsing is considered a normal phase of behaviour change, especially for those people who are trying a particular change for the first time. It is important for the health promoter to convey to the client that relapsing can act as a positive learning experience. It is rare that people succeed the first time around with any behaviour change, but lessons will have been learnt which can prove invaluable during the next attempt. The client may wish to take a break and try again another time. The health promoter needs to leave the door open and encourage them to try again at a future date. Figure 7.2 shows an example of using the model to recognise the stages of change in an individual pursuing weight loss.

Social Prescribing

This is the means whereby health promoters use community resources to help individuals with behaviour change. This may mean referrals to community gyms, allotment schemes, exercise on prescription, cook and eat courses, befriending schemes and a range of other services which may be available within reach. Although social prescribing has been part of the UK's health promotion strategies for some years now, the lack of robust evidence to prove its worth in increasing the health and well-being of individuals undertaking various activities means that this strategy has yet to be proven (Bickerdike et al. 2017). Despite the problems with a firm evidence base of effectiveness, these schemes are popular with those who are referred to them and continue to be utilised as a key health promotion resource, especially as a way of improving mental health and tackling social isolation.

Digital and Mobile Health Behaviour Interventions

As previously discussed, there is a growing prevalence of digital and mobile apps and de-vices to aid people with behaviour change. These take the form of text messages, apps, wearable devices or websites. In 2020, NICE published its review of research into the use and effectiveness of this technology in helping with behaviour change. It concluded that there was inconsistent and insufficient evidence that the use of such technology was effective and should be used instead of other services. Most of the existing research did not compare

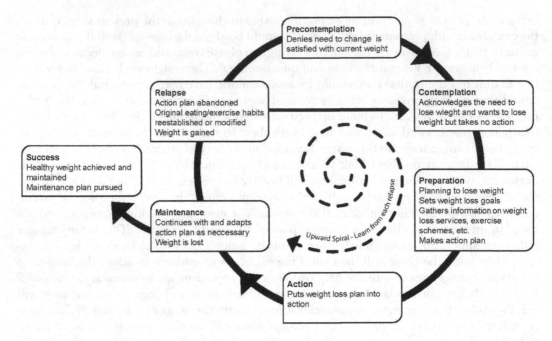

Figure 7.2 Adaptation of Prochaska and DiClemente's (1984) Transtheoretical Model to Show Stages of Change for Clients Undertaking Weight Loss

digital interventions with current practice. Therefore, NICE does not recommend replacement of existing evidence-based services with digital at the present time (National Institute for Health and Care Excellence (NICE) 2020). However, it acknowledged that digital and mobile devices may be of use for those individuals who were unable to access face-to-face consultations. It may be just early days in these innovations with more higher quality research needed into the effectiveness of such devices, and evidence-based technology may become a useful partner in the future as long as they are checked for safety and data security.

Motivational Interviewing (MI)

Motivational Interviewing is another tried and tested approach in the field of behaviour change. It has proven to be particularly effective when working with the ambivalent or multivalent clients, those in the pre-contemplative or early contemplative stages of change, where the motivation for change appears to be either very low or at best 'hanging in the balance', thus holding the client in a position of inertia or 'stuck-ness' (Motivational Interviewing Network of Trainers (MINT) 2022).

Background

MI is an empirically supported, testable clinical approach to facilitating constructive and helpful conversations about change. It first emerged in 1983 in an article written by its originator Dr. William R. Miller (Miller 1983) and was presented as an alternative approach to the prevailing culture in the addictions field at that time. This traditional approach consisted of a coercive and confrontational style, intent on inundating people with harsh facts and poor prognosis data as a means of trying to bring about the changes deemed necessary in the best interest of their recovery. Since the early 1990s, in partnership with Dr. Stephen Rollnick, MI evolved and developed into an authoritative, strongly evidence-based approach to resolving the common challenges faced by those involved in the field of behaviour change work. Clients can present to professionals at a point in their life or stage of change where they have recognised that there is a problem and have in some way acknowledged that 'something does indeed need to change'. They may have knocked on the door of a health professional and willingly asked for help. Even so, the health promoter's journey with most clients is likely to encounter some pressure points and obstacles along the way towards the proposed change goal. The challenge is likely to be much greater with clients who are less ready, willing and/ or able to make changes, for example, those who have been sent to services by a third party. This may be a family doctor or a concerned parent or partner, or because a certain set of unexpected circumstances have arisen (e.g. a recent health scare, accident or acute episode, an unplanned pregnancy, an arrest for a drunk driving offence or possession of illegal substances). Whilst for some people such events may serve as a catalyst or prompt for change, others may not be at a stage of recognition and acknowledgement at all. They may even be resentful, offended or angry about the intervention and could almost certainly be described as change averse, pre-contemplative or ambivalent about behaviour change. This discord or oppositional position can manifest itself in negative client body language, poor attendance at services and increased levels of anti-change language, termed 'sustain speech'. Client utterances such as: 'Yes but'; 'I've tried that before and it didn't work'; 'Everyone is just making too much of a big deal out of this'; 'All my friends drink as much as I do and no-one is giving them a hard time'; 'Well have *you* ever had this problem?'; 'It never did her any harm ...' etc. Today, research continues to demonstrate that when met with such client ambivalence or opposition, many practitioners will resort to providing them with what they seem to be 'lacking', that is, unsolicited advice, information, knowledge, imposed insight or skills associated with the issue in question. This is provided with the well intentioned aim of using a good argument to 'convince' them to change for their own good, yet this often has a very limited positive effect. MI offers, instead, a way of eliciting from people *their own* thoughts, concerns, views and ideas about change, so motivation is *evoked* rather than installed. It builds on the belief that an overly directive practitioner style is counterproductive when indecision and reluctance (termed ambivalence) are observed in the client and may engender counterchange (sustain speech) or an oppositional stance from the client. MI conversations can vary in length from very brief, just a few informal minutes, to longer therapeutic sessions of an hour or so. They can take place with individuals or groups from a diverse range of ages and backgrounds and across a broad range of subject areas, homogeneous and heterogeneous. The MI practitioner's attitude is always one of warmth, openness and genuine compassionate curiosity about the client's dilemma, coupled with a gentle guiding approach to encourage them to move forward. The practitioner aims to cultivate a respectful and collaborative environment within which client receptivity and readiness for change can be skilfully explored and increased (Motivational Interviewing UK and Ireland 2022). 'It is designed to strengthen an individual's motivation for and movement toward a specific goal by eliciting and exploring the person's own reasons for change within an atmosphere of acceptance and compassion' (Miller and Rollnick 2012, p. 5).

How Does MI Work?

MI is a strengths-based approach which utilises a four-process model – 1) Engage, 2) Focus, 3) Evoke and 4) Plan – in conjunction with a core set of person-centred micro-skills

(OARS) – Open Questions, Affirmations, Reflections and Summaries. These fundamental components are skilfully woven together and imbued with the qualities of compassion, acceptance, partnership and empowerment (Spirit) to support and *guide* people towards resolving their own change dilemma and to develop a commitment to their own change goal. There is a particular focus on the language of change and commitment (Change Talk) and the practitioner skilfully endeavours to evoke and increase the quantity and strength of genuine change talk expressed by the client by mindfully avoiding the traps that encourage defensiveness and counter-change/sustain language (the latter of which is shown to decrease the likelihood of change outcomes).

The **Four Processes** are both sequential and recursive in nature, rather than worked through in rigid stages or phases. They form a semi structured framework or sort of compass bearing or reference point for the flow and direction of the MI conversation.

1 **Engage** – Therapeutic engagement or a positive practitioner–client relationship is seen as a necessary precursor to all that follows. The quality of the relationship as rated by the client is a strong predictor of retention and outcome. Engagement is necessary throughout the intervention and not simply at the outset.
2 **Focus** – Leading naturally from engaging to a spotlight on a particular agenda, i.e. what the person came to talk about, balanced with some things the practitioner may need to raise or cover. This is a collaborative process of clarifying and agreeing on the direction of travel and what the change hopes/targets/goals are for the session(s).
3 **Evoke** – This is at the heart of MI and involves drawing from the client their own ideas about why and how they might go about making the change. It is the opposite to being expert-led or directive and utilises the client's own wisdom and insight at the core of the intervention.
4 **Plan** – This is when readiness for change builds to a tipping point and the energy subtly shifts towards the 'how, where and when' of change and away from the 'why' of change. Planning encompasses both the development of an action plan and a commitment to carrying through with the plan. (A plan without commitment is not a strong indicator of change.)

The Micro-skills OARS

These are the conduit for excellent person-centred communication as it is through the skilful use of these elements that the entire MI conversation takes place.

- **Open Questions** – Used to open up and encourage conversation flow, evoke an expression of the client's thoughts and insights and minimise short one-word answers where possible. They usually begin, 'How might you....' 'Tell me about....' 'What are your thoughts on....' etc. In general, practitioners tend to rely heavily on questions and in MI there is much more reliance on the use of reflection (see below). A ratio of one question to two or three reflections is a useful guide for an MI conversation.
- **Affirmations** – Statements of validation or confirmation usually about strengths, values, qualities, efforts, etc. that the practitioner has noticed in the client and offered to them in the form of a reflective verbal 'gift'. Research shows that effective affirmation leads to an increase in client change talk (see below). Tips for good affirmation include being genuine – don't offer it if you don't mean it; specific rather than general, e.g. 'you have made a big effort not to smoke in the same room as the children' rather than 'you've been trying hard'; and to use it sparingly where it will have the most impact (like seasoning in food – it can be overused!) (Miller and Moyers 2017).

- **Reflections** – By far, the communication skill is used most frequently and strategically by the MI practitioner. Reflections can be simple, sticking closely to the words used by the client, or more complex where the practitioner aims to be more interpretive by imagining walking in the client's shoes or by using a range of specific reflection strategies to encourage particular responses, e.g. use of a double-sided reflection to illuminate the ambivalence which is keeping the client stuck. For example, the practitioner may say, 'so on the one hand you really enjoy cooking and entertaining and holding parties, and on the other you are feeling increasingly unhappy about the way your weight is affecting your confidence in social situations'. A good reflection encourages the client to reach inside and share more of their internal world, like holding a mirror up to their expressed thoughts, which can really help them explore and gain a deeper understanding of their dilemma. Tips for good reflection include trying to avoid the use of lots of sentence stems such as 'So it sounds like....' 'It seems like you may be saying...' 'So....' 'I think I'm right in hearing you say...', etc. It is generally preferable to use less of this type of 'therapy' language and keep the flow more conversational in style. Also, it is not necessary to tag an open question onto the end of every reflection. Try to trust the process and let the reflection resonate with the client.
- **Summaries** – Offered periodically throughout the conversation as a means of providing punctuation and pace and demonstrating accurate listening to the client. These are used strategically to emphasise and possibly link certain relevant themes and to re-emphasise important elements such as client change talk statements. Summaries are also used strategically to encourage a gentle forward direction to the conversation and to avoid repetition and 'going around in circles'. Tips for summaries include keeping it simple – less is often more, and you do not need to include everything in a summary!

Information and Advice Giving in MI

Due to the person-centred nature of the micro-skills (OARS) and the Spirit, many practitioners mistakenly interpret MI as an approach which does not allow for the giving of information or advice. This is not the case as MI is both person-centred and goal-oriented. What is important, however, is the when and how of this type of exchange. A useful format – Elicit, Provide, Elicit (E-P-E) – has been developed to help keep the process within MI 'territory' by asking permission to share and assuming that people have knowledge and insight that should be 'mined' before bringing in any additional information. This style of exchange helps us avoid the expert trap – i.e. I am right and you are wrong. Below is an example of an interaction using MI techniques.

Activity

You are a health visitor, discussing childhood immunisations with a mother at a baby clinic. How would you gauge and respond to the mother's anxiety regarding vaccinating her child?

Mother: I don't like the idea of having him vaccinated.
        It may be tempting to jump in and provide information about the benefits of vaccination. Instead, like in any nursing intervention, there is first the need to assess. Anxieties, expectations and information the mother already holds need to be elicited.

Health Visitor:	'So tell me what you've heard about the baby immunisation programme?' (First **Elicit**)
Mother:	'It sometimes goes wrong doesn't it? I mean you don't know what's in that stuff, or if it will cause more harm than good, it's not natural'.
	Rather than contradicting the mother, the health visitor seeks to understand and respect her anxieties, affirming her concerns.
Health Visitor:	'You have been really thinking about what's best for your baby, and you want to do the right thing' (*Empathic Reflection*).
Mother:	'Well I've read stuff about it causing disabilities in certain children and I don't want to risk that'.
Health Visitor:	'You have read some worrying things and it sounds like there are some specific concerns that you'd like to explore to help you make the best decision' (*Reflection*).
Health Visitor:	'I could go through some of the information about why we encourage immunisation in babies, including some of the potential risks, to see what you think?' (*Asking permission to provide information*).
	The health visitor then presents information in a *neutral* fashion, using prefixes such as 'what the research has shown', 'what other parents have said', etc., rather than 'I think you should' or 'What you need to do is....'
Health Visitor:	What do you make of that? What are your thoughts at this point? (Final **Elicit**)
	This final elicit is designed to check out understanding and allows the parent to agree or disagree with the information without it seeming like a personal disagreement, thus maintaining the client-practitioner relationship. It is most important not to pressurise. The client needs time and space to consider. However, providing written information, details of websites, etc. may be useful to help her with the decision. If the mother is unable to reach a decision at this point, the Health Visitor can follow this up at a later date.

The Ethos or Key Principles of MI

- **Spirit** – A set of values or ethics which serve as a reminder that MI is not simply a box of tools or techniques, 'but a way of being with and for people, the mind-set and heart-set from which one practices MI' (Rollnick and Miller 1995). The following four points go some way to encompassing the empowering intention of this essential aspect of MI.
- **Partnership** – MI is something that is carried out collaboratively with and for others and not something which is imposed, inflicted or 'done to' them. The practitioner makes every effort to reduce the inevitable power dynamic that exists between 'professional' and 'client' by relating to them as another human being, and by exploring, acknowledging and respecting the expertise that they bring from their own life and experiences.
- **Acceptance** – It is subdivided into four categories: Absolute Worth, Autonomy, Accurate Empathy, and Affirmation. In summary, 'taken together, these four person centred

conditions convey what we mean by acceptance. One honours each person's *absolute worth* and potential as a human being, recognises and supports the person's irrevocable *autonomy* to choose his or her own way, seeks through *accurate empathy* to understand the other's perspective, and *affirms* the person's strengths and efforts' (Miller and Roll-nick 2012).

- **Compassion** – A genuine desire for the well-being of others, this is not just about being nice and kind but is 'the wish to see others free from suffering' (Dalai Lama 2013). The practitioner actively prioritises the needs and welfare of the client.
- **Evocation** – The strengths-based approach to eliciting answers and solutions from the client. This is based on the belief that most people have the necessary internal resources to resolve their issues, especially with a little help to draw them forth, rather than on a deficit model which looks for shortcomings so that these can be corrected or re-installed from the expert position.

Change Talk

Change Talk is perceived in a unique way in Motivational Interviewing. It refers to the language of change as expressed by the client during the session and is significantly linked to the prediction of the outcome. The MI practitioner intentionally seeks to encourage and increase levels of genuine client change talk by utilising all of the aforementioned skills and avoiding traps which may incur the elicitation of sustained talk (language which supports the status quo). Change talk can be considered in two phases, The Preparatory Phase and The Mobilising Phase. The first category includes Desire, Ability, Reason and Need for change (DARN) and is more prevalent during the earlier stages of change, i.e. when ambivalence is still a significant feature of the conversation.

1) Preparatory Change Talk (DARN)

- **Desire** for change, e.g. 'I *wish* I was fit enough to go running with my friend'.
- **Ability** to change, e.g. 'I think I *could* give up smoking if I put my mind to it'.
- **Reason(s)** for change, e.g. 'I want to lose weight to *look good for my wedding* in 6 months'.
- **Need** for change, e.g. 'With my family history of breast cancer, I really *need* to cut my drinking right down'.

The second phase comes into place as ambivalence is resolving and there is an increase in momentum and volition towards the change goal. It includes Commitment, Activation and Taking Steps (CAT). It is important that an MI practitioner can recognise, elicit and respond to change talk as well as differentiate between the categories in order to adjust their response accordingly. Missing the opportunity to shift gear when a client has subtly indicated a nudge towards change can result in a decline in their motivation.

2) Mobilising Change Talk (CAT)

- **Commitment** to change, e.g. 'I *will* start going to the quit smoking group next week', 'I *promise*....', 'I *am* definitely going to...', etc.
- **Activation** – signs of being ready, willing and able, preparing for change
- **Taking Steps** – evidence and examples of change beginning/happening in current time frame.

Research has shown that when sufficient and appropriately matched attention is given to client DARN language (usually in the form of reflection, affirmation or evocative questioning), a corresponding increase in CAT language is observed, indicating an enhanced likelihood of actual change.

Key Messages

- Health professionals should opportunistically raise the issue of behaviour change with their clients.
- When considering behaviour change, people weigh up the costs and benefits of what the change will mean to them.
- It is important that practitioners are aware of services and techniques which can support clients through behaviour change and these are discussed with rather than imposed on clients.
- Some clients are able to instigate and maintain behaviour change themselves, while others require more support.
- Supporting people who find behaviour change difficult requires in-depth assessment of their ability and motivation to change. This exploratory conversation and relationship building is key and needs time.
- A person-centred approach which is affirmative of clients' actions is much more likely to be effective than a directive approach, 'being with' clients rather than 'doing to' clients.
- It is important to work with the client's experience, skills and knowledge of themselves and their circumstances to formulate solutions rather than imposing solutions on them.
- Motivational Interviewing is a useful series of techniques which can be used to support clients who are ambivalent regarding behaviour change.
- Positive change talk used by the client, especially commitment language, is a strong predictor of actual change.

References

Bhattacharya, A., Kolovson, S., Sung, Y.-C., Eacker, M., Chen, M., Munson, S.A. and Kientz, J.A. (2018). Understanding pivotal experiences in behavior change for the design of technologies for personal wellbeing. *Journal of Biomedical Informatics* [online], 79, pp. 129–142. doi: 10.1016/j.jbi.2018.01.002.

Bickerdike, L., Booth, A., Wilson, P.M., Farley, K. and Wright, K. (2017). Social prescribing: Less rhetoric and more reality. A systematic review of the evidence. *BMJ Open* [online], 7(4), p. e013384. doi: 10.1136/bmjopen-2016-013384.

Bmj.com. (2020). *Healthy habits in middle age linked to longer life free from disease | BMJ* [online]. Available at: https://www.bmj.com/company/newsroom/healthy-habits-in-middle-age-linked-to-longer-life-free-from-disease/

Cochrane Collaboration. (2008). *Physician advice for smoking cessation (review)*. London: Wiley and Sons.

Dalai Lama. (2013). *Teachings*. Available at: http://www.dalailama.com/teachings/training-the-mind/verse-2

Department of Health. (2010). *Healthy lives, healthy people. Our strategy for public health in England*. London: Department of Health.

Dosh, S., Holtrop, J., Torres, T., Arnold, A., Bauman, J. and White, L. (2005). Changing organizational constructs into functional tools: An assessment of the 5 A's in primary care practices. *Annals of Family Medicine*, 3(Suppl 2), pp. 50–52.

Haighton, C., Newbury-Birch, D., Durlik, C., Sallis, A., Chadborn, T., Porter, L., Harling, M. and Rodrigues, A. (2021). Optimizing making every contact count (MECC) interventions: A strategic behavioral analysis. *Health Psychology* [online], 40(12), pp. 960–973. doi: 10.1037/hea0001100.

Martínez, C., Castellano, Y., Andrés, A., Fu, M., Antón, L., Ballbè, M., Fernández, P., Cabrera, S., Riccobene, A., Gavilan, E., Feliu, A., Baena, A., Margalef, M. and Fernández, E. (2017). Factors associated with implementation of the 5A's smoking cessation model. *Tobacco Induced Diseases* [online], 15(1). doi: 10.1186/s12971-017-0146-7.

Miller, W.R. (1983). Motivational interviewing with problem drinkers. *Behavioural Psychotherapy*, 11, pp. 147–172.

Miller, W.R. and Moyers, T.B. (2017). Motivational interviewing and the clinical science of Carl Rogers. *Journal of Consulting and Clinical Psychology*, 85(8), pp. 757–766.

Miller, W.R. and Rollnick, S. (2012). *Motivational interviewing – Helping people change.* 3rd ed. Guilford: Guilford Press.

Motivational Interviewing Network of Trainers (MINT). (2022). *Motivational interviewing network of trainers.* Available at: www.motivationalinter viewing.org

Motivational Interviewing UK and Ireland. (2022). *What is MI?* [online] Available at: https://www. mintukandireland.org/what-is-mi.html

NHS Future Forum. (2010). *The NHS's role in the public's health.* London: Department of Health.

National Institute for Health and Care Excellence (NICE). (2020). *Behaviour change: Digital and mobile health interventions guideline* [online]. Available at: https://www.nice.org.uk/guidance/ng183/resources/behaviour-change-digital-and-mobile-health-interventions-pdf-66142020002245

Nutbeam, D. and Harris, E. (2004). *Theory in a nutshell: A practical guide to health promotion theories.* Sydney, NSW: McGraw-Hill.

Prochaska, J. and DiClemente, C. (1984). The transtheoretical approach: Crossing traditional boundaries of change. Homewood: Dow Jones/Irwin.

Rollnick, S. and Miller, W.R. (1995). What is motivational interviewing? *Behavioural and Cognitive Psychotherapy*, 23, pp. 325–334.

Rosenstock I.M., Strecher V.J. and Becker M.H. (1988) Social learning theory and the health belief model. *Health Education Behaviour* 15(2), pp. 175–183.

Schunk, D.H. and DiBenedetto, M.K. (2021). Self-efficacy and human motivation. *Advances in Motivation Science* [online], pp. 153–179. doi: 10.1016/bs.adms.2020.10.001.

Simply Psychology.org. (2022). *Extrinsic vs. intrinsic motivation: What's the difference?* [online] Available at: https://simplypsychology.org/differences-between-extrinsic-and-intrinsic-motivation.html

Swanson, V. and Maltinsky, W. (2019). Motivational and behaviour change approaches for improving diabetes management. *Practical Diabetes* [online], 36(4), pp. 121–125. doi: 10.1002/pdi.2229.

8 Programme Planning

Susan R. Thompson, Jane Bethea
and Oliver Wilkinson-Dale

Levels of Intervention

Public health programmes tend to be categorised in terms of primary, secondary and tertiary prevention programmes. Primary prevention programmes are designed to tackle the determinants or causes of certain conditions in order to prevent those conditions from occurring. There are many such interventions in place to do this and such interventions form much of the focus of the work of health promoters and primary health care professionals. Tackling obesity in order to prevent CVD and diabetes, for instance, and providing free condoms and sexual health advice to reduce sexually transmitted diseases are just two examples. Secondary prevention is work done in order to prevent an existing condition from worsening. Giving medication or performing coronary angioplasty to patients with angina to stop their condition from proceeding to a heart attack is such an example. Tertiary prevention is preventing the complications of an existing condition. For example, people with diabetes are at risk of developing diabetic retinopathy and also poor circulation, which may lead to leg ulcers and poor healing ability. It is important, therefore, that their blood sugar levels are carefully controlled and are given regular monitoring appointments to screen for such complications and given advice regarding appropriate self-care so that risks may be reduced. Health services engage in all three levels of prevention, but other agencies such as local authorities and the voluntary sector are more able to be involved in primary prevention than secondary or tertiary prevention. However, organisations such as patient groups and voluntary agencies may be involved (certainly in providing information) at all three levels.

Interventions also vary in intrusiveness. Some low level or potential future health issues are just monitored with no other interventions being proposed. Interventions range from this low level monitoring, to providing specific information regarding certain risk factors, then incentives and disincentives for individual behaviour change and, finally, restricting or legislating to try to completely eliminate an unhealthy choice which is seen to detrimentally impact health, banning the sale of tobacco products to those under 18, for example. These different levels of interventions are illustrated in the Nuffield Council on Bioethics (2007) (Figure 8.1). The level of intervention proposed is dependent on the number of people affected, the seriousness of the health issue and the cost of it to the economy and health services.

Legislation, which is the highest level of intervention, is rarely resorted to. Mostly governments prefer to work with manufacturers to set industry guidelines and agreements aimed at limiting damage. However, the childhood obesity crisis and the fact that children, especially those from a poorer background, get so much of their calories from high sugar soft drinks (American Institute for Cancer Research 2020; World Health Organization [WHO] 2017) resulted in the UK government introducing a sugar tax in 2018. This imposed a tax

DOI: 10.4324/9781003411321-8

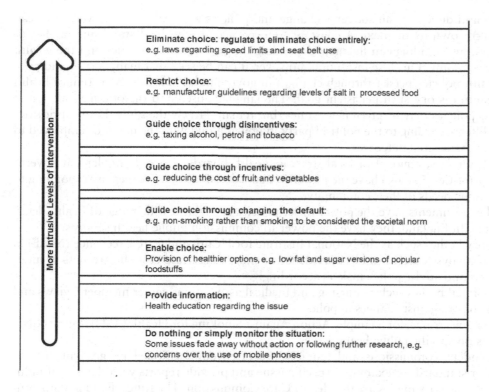

Figure 8.1 The Intervention Ladder (Nuffield Council on Bioethics 2007)

on drinks which contain more than 5 g sugar per 100 ml, thereby making those drinks more expensive to buy. The aim of the tax was to encourage manufacturers to reduce their output of high sugar drinks and switch to low calorie drink production instead. This has been successful with output of high sugar drinks now comprising just 15% of the market share, compared with a massive 50% prior to the imposition of the tax (Bmj.com 2021). More recently, again with the aim of reducing obesity, the UK government has required restaurants and other food outlets to state the calorific content of the meals they are serving, placing these on menus so that customers are better informed, with the hope that they may choose less calorific options (GOV.UK 2022a). It seems that the UK government at least is now more inclined than in previous years to legislate the food industry, rather than relying on industry guidelines which have not impacted the growing obesity crisis.

Policy Makers

Given below is a list of the main public and private bodies that set or contribute to public health policies.

- Government health departments and health ministers. Although links are complex, research has shown that those countries which are democratic, have welfare provision, high public spending and less inequalities generally have populations with better health than those countries that do not have these elements (McCartney et al. 2019). Policies are strongly influenced by the ethos of the political party in power, which means health policy and direction can suddenly change and policies adopted by one government can be overthrown by the next. A constant 'reform' agenda can be destabilising for health services, and funding can fluctuate depending on government priorities and the wealth of the economy. On close inspection, however, it can be seen that many health and public health policies persist through changes in governments. The policy to reduce health inequalities is one such persistent goal. The language used and rhetoric may alter, and similar policies may be given new names, but remain largely the same. Health priorities may differ according to the political party in power along with the methods employed to achieve the desired outcomes.

- Health services, regional or local strategic health boards, generally implement government priorities, but also have the power to make decisions that are seen as responding to the specific needs of their community.
- Local governments have the power to set policies to tackle a wide range of health determinants. In England, they have the power to commission public health services.
- Advisory bodies such as the National Institute for Health and Care Excellence (NICE) in the UK analyse current research, evidence of effectiveness and cost-effectiveness of interventions and advise policy makers accordingly.
- Professional bodies such as nursing and medical associations gather members' views and lobby for or against changes in policy.
- Single issue groups, for example, Action Against Smoking for Health (ASH), lobby policy makers on specific public health issues.
- Independent commissions and inquires are often commissioned by governments to monitor standards or examine a specific issue and provide reports with the aim of influencing policy. Examples are the Health Care Commission, The King's Fund and government inquires into specific problem services that have been found to fall short of the care needed.

Risk Versus Benefit Analysis

Public health services generally use data regarding known associations or causes and effects to decide on programmes which target certain individuals and communities considered at high risk of developing certain diseases, injuries or social issues. This is seen as a cost-effective use of resources, for example, the individual calculation of CVD risk and the subsequent treatment regimens discussed in Chapter 2. Certain at-risk populations are also targeted. Young people truanting from school are at greater risk of developing a drug habit than their more affluent peers (Drug Education Forum 2013). So, preventative services may be set up targeted at these individuals and not others. Another benefit of targeting high-risk populations is that both staff and client motivation may be high as the intervention is seen as relevant to the client group and the benefit versus risk ratio is higher (Davies and Macdowall 2006). Alternatively, an approach which includes the whole of the population may be seen as wasteful as many of those targeted will not gain a benefit. The Framingham Coronary Heart Disease study showed that if all men up to the age of 55 years reduced their cholesterol levels by 10%, one man in 50 would avoid a heart attack but that the remaining 49 would have eaten a healthier diet without actually needing to (Rose 1992). When statistics such as one man in 50 are scaled up to a population level, the actual numbers are impressive and significant enough for governments and health services to try to reduce the cost of such diseases. However, the cost for the individual is high. The risk of a woman contracting HIV from an infected partner during unprotected penile-vaginal intercourse is one in a thousand (Centers for Disease Control and Prevention [CDC] 2013), yet the risk is probably perceived to be much higher due to the publicity of the safe sex message and the profile of HIV in the public's consciousness. Public health is about ensuring the best possible health for the population, but in order to achieve this, the risks for the individual are often overemphasised.

The Planning Cycle

The first stage of programme planning is to establish a need and hence a rationale for instigating a programme in the first place. As seen in Chapter 5, health needs assessment can take many forms and when completed, the results of needs assessments are used to formulate the strategic plans of organisations which consider policies and programmes to address the needs identified and prioritised. Strategic plans should encompass all agencies that have a responsibility or influence with regard to the issue in question. This 'joined up working' ensures that different aspects of the need are addressed and that all partner organisations work towards common goals. Table 8.1 gives examples of how different agencies may contribute to improving road safety, a primary prevention intervention.

Programme planning involves getting together many different agencies, organisations and client groups for discussions, and the logistics of this is difficult in itself. Different agencies have different planning cycles and different priorities for funding and action. Therefore, it is essential that a consensus is reached and sources of finance are identified and committed by each agency with roles made clear. A crucial point is that commitment comes from executive heads at the top of each organisation and only then will commitment to action and funding result. Difficulties may emerge following a change of management and, therefore, priorities. This should be guarded against to ensure sustainability. Time scales need to be kept, if at all possible, to prevent slippage and the project drifting. There are many planning models, for example, Ewles and Simnett (2017) and Nutbeam, Harris and Wise (2010), but most have a similar basic format and follow a logical process (see Figures 8.2 and 8.3). Following a recognised model ensures that programmes have a good chance of being effective and all relevant information is taken into account. Good planning focuses on the achievement of agreed outcomes, makes workers prioritise and justify their activities and enables the pursuit and evaluation of an action plan.

Planning a Programme Aimed at Reducing Illegal Drug Use

Suppose it has been decided that there is a need to tackle the level of illegal drug use within a particular locality. Firstly, the level of the issue should be established by accessing epidemiological and demographic information. Statistics regarding the use of certain drugs, such as

Table 8.1 Agencies and Actions Working Together to Improve Road Safety

Agency	Action
Police	Prosecution of driving offences, speed cameras
Highways Agency	Speed bumps, 20 miles/h zone near schools,
Education Authority	pedestrian crossings
Driving Standards Authority	School bus provision, school crossing patrols
Parent Groups	Set standards for driver competence
	Organise volunteer walk to school schemes

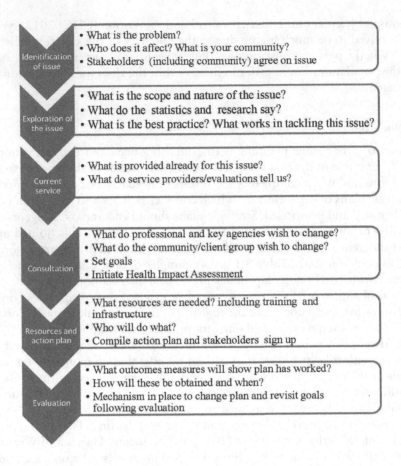

Figure 8.2 Programme Planning

heroin and crack cocaine, are collected by services and by public health observatories. It is also important to look at the trends over time. Are incidence rates increasing or decreasing? Possibly, if they are decreasing at a satisfactory rate, there is no need to change the current plan. Key stakeholders, both lay and professional, need to be approached by the organisation taking the lead to ascertain potential involvement in any future project. There should be consultation with local people via community workers or partnership organisations with the question asked as to whether drug misuse is a concern to the local population, professionals and voluntary organisations in the area. Ideally, issues to be acted upon should be a priority for the local people, not just for health care organisations and the government. A review of the research regarding the determinants or causes of illegal drug use should be undertaken as root causes will need to be addressed if programmes are to be at all effective. The use of heroin and crack cocaine is often both a cause and a consequence of social exclusion and is more common in areas with high unemployment, poor housing standards and amongst the homeless population (Atkins 2018). Next, it is useful to examine evidence from past programmes of intervention, locally and nationally and possibly internationally for similar populations. What seems to have been evaluated well and appears to have had some success? In the UK, the following fit this criterion: drug prevention activities, assessments of those at risk and provision of tailor-made skills training for these young people

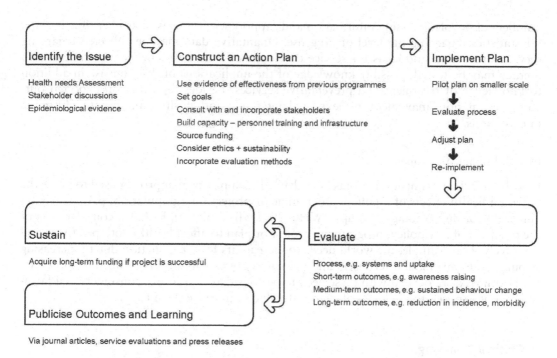

Figure 8.3 Project Planning in Health Promotion and Public Health

and adults, funding for and greater access to treatment services (GOV.UK 2022b; Nice. org.uk 2017). Such initiatives should be considered with the logistics, funding and sustainability issues taken into account. The capacity of various stakeholders to contribute should be ascertained and commitment agreed. Consultation on possible action plans should be undertaken with the wider community and local workers. Resources should be identified including the funding required and the cost-effectiveness of interventions considered. Also needed to be considered are what workers are available, professionals or lay people, what their training needs may be and what infrastructure will be required, such as venues for proposed services. It is useful to garner political and community support for the programme from key community figures and local government representatives who will champion the programme, raising awareness and guaranteeing give backing for the programme's initiatives. Health impact assessments need to be carried out (see below) and a pilot planned so initiatives can be tried out and lessons learnt. Evaluation is the key and needs to be in place from the very start and during every stage of the programme to establish whether goals have been met. Evaluations are essential if funding is to be secured to sustain the programme into the future and will be required to be rigorous to pass the stringent tests for cost-effectiveness from the various funding bodies supporting the programme. However, the nature of health promotion programmes fails to lend themselves to randomised controlled trials which are considered to be the gold standard by which effectiveness within the medical field is proved. Evaluation should use both quantitative and qualitative methods and consider process and short-, medium- and long-term outcomes (Nutbeam 1999; O'Connor-Fleming et al. 2006; Public Health England 2018; WHO 2001). As most action plans are multifaceted, with many interventions targeted at different aspects of the problem, evaluations need to follow suit. Quantitative statistics regarding drug misuse interventions may consist of recording numbers of people accessing information and support services as well as over time looking for statistics regarding the level of drug use. Qualitative data may be collected regarding service satisfaction and ideas for service development from both clients and staff. Health literacy may be tested, possibly knowledge of the implications of drug misuse in addition to knowledge of treatment and preventative services. Besides reporting on expected outcomes, evaluations may uncover unexpected outcomes, both positive and negative from the interventions.

Health Impact Assessment

Health impact assessment (HIA) has been defined as 'a practical approach used to judge the potential health effects of a policy, programme or project on a population, particularly on vulnerable or disadvantaged groups' (WHO 2022). Basically, an HIA is a consideration of the potential of any policy, programme, project or plan to affect health, both positively and negatively. For example, the world needs to increase its food production due to increasing population numbers, and fertilisers and pesticides are essential tools to do this. However, the health risks associated with these need to be considered to ensure consumers and farmers are not exposed to the levels of chemicals which can cause them harm.

Critical Thinking

Take some time out to think about the following:

There is a proposal for opening a factory in a suburban area. What might its impact be on the local community and what might be the benefits or disadvantages?

Many negative results of policies are indirect. This proposal may be considered to be a good thing for the local economy and jobs, but it will also probably increase traffic congestion and pollution.

The resulting increase in traffic may cause an increase in road traffic accidents. More vehicle traffic also causes an increase in pollution levels and subsequently worsening respiratory illnesses. Will the jobs actually fit the skill set of local workers? Or, will the workers travel into the area?

The combination of the above would make the factory deliver negative outcomes for the local community with little, if any, positives.

Equity is a key value that should be considered when undertaking an HIA as most proposals benefit some people at the cost of others.

It is important for key stakeholders to be consulted and for both long-term and short-term impacts considered. HIA attempts to predict positive and negative outcomes that may result from proposed policies or programmes and to try and mitigate these (Flowers and Evans 2020). To do this, it is important that good quality evidence is available to programme planners so that predictions will be as accurate as possible. These predictions may be based on the experience of similar programmes or policies in similar areas (Kemm 2001). The difficulty is that policies and programmes are complex and diverse and sometimes competing.

HIAs seek to way up the balance of harm versus benefit and are essential if policy impacts are to be understood, harm lessened and overall benefits increased. HIA has a broad reach. HIAs are conducted on proposals as diverse as the sighting of a new supermarket to global mining consortiums needing to ensure that their industry is seen to be ethical and responsible. HIAs need to be conducted at the early planning stage to enable proposals to be modified in light of their recommendations so that health can be safeguarded and enhanced (Birley 2011). As a health promoter, you may be directly involved in HIAs for specific health or non-health projects. For example, you may be involved in consultation with the community to be affected, an essential stage in gathering evidence regarding potential impact. The WHO provides a website which gives examples of HIAs and suggests tools for policy makers to use in order to undertake HIAs when planning policies and programmes (WHO 2022).

Working with Communities to Plan Interventions

A community may be defined as a body of people joined together by a common denominator. This may be by living in the same geographical community, having a particular medical condition or social need or a set of circumstances which bind people together. Community profiling or assessing the needs of a particular community is an important first step in working with communities. The information gained from questionnaires, focus groups, social networks, voluntary organisations and neighbourhood groups is essential to achieve a picture of the perceived needs of the community in focus. This primary data married to the secondary epidemiological data and evidence gained from local authorities and health and social care services can create a complete picture of that community.

In addition to identifying needs, it is important to consider the resources present in the community, its assets, strengths and existing service provision. This is important to establish before planning projects and initiatives. It also prevents profiles from focusing entirely on unmet needs which can be both distorting and demoralising (Hawtin and Percy-Smith 2007). When considering workers who will deliver different aspects of the programme, it is again important to consider the potential or existing skills present in the community in question. This prevents the 'top down' approach of outside professionals swooping in and 'doing to' communities. Whether it be a neighbourhood community or one connected by a common issue, individuals in that community will possess valuable insight and knowledge of issues which will not be possessed by outsiders. Utilising these skills, for example, by the use of peer educators can give the project credibility within the community and provide personal development opportunities for the workers in question. Peer education has been shown to be especially effective with younger people around sexual health and mental health and supporting women with breastfeeding. It is important that peer educators themselves are supported within a robust organisational framework (Tolli 2012; Topping 2022). Hopefully, through involvement in projects, peer educators will benefit from increased health literacy and self-esteem (Asthana and Halliday 2006). Individuals within communities vary in their engagement with each other and their willingness to be involved in the life of their community. This level of community resource is termed social capital and although a complex and abstract concept, tools have been devised to measure it. Indicators for social capital include the level of trust in a community, engagement in volunteering, voter turnout and membership of community organisations. Research has shown that high levels of social capital result in better mental and physical health within a community (Ehsan et al. 2019). The more public involvement and commitment to projects, the greater the chance

of successful interventions. Involvement of the community and a comprehensive needs assessment are used to inform the planning of initiatives and projects and are usually a pre-
requisite for funding applications. However, gaining input and true representation from a
local community, client group or service users is often easier said than done. There can also
be negative effects on active individuals within the community, some of whom may feel the
burden of representing the community, whilst others may feel that their views are not being
taken into account, so care is needed (Villalonga-Olives and Kawachi 2017). The first step is
to gather together a group of interested parties or stakeholders. For a geographical locality,
this may be local residents, statutory and voluntary local service providers, local businesses
and local councillors. For a specific issue, this may be service users and carers, statutory and
voluntary agencies and academic experts. The steering group needs to set parameters and
terms of reference for the group, for example, geographical boundaries, age ranges, clients
with certain characteristics, diagnosis, etc. It is important to have key players on the steering group, those people who have valuable knowledge of the politics (with a small 'p') and
history of the community and previous efforts at intervention. This hopefully will highlight
sensitivities and limit the risk of blundering in and subsequently alienating the target group.
Community development workers, local neighbourhood workers or project workers are
an essential resource in this regard. Such volunteers or workers hopefully have developed
enough local knowledge and trust within the community to have a 'way in' to key influ-
ential community figures and therefore access to the wider community. The knowledge of
specific local circumstances and power politics involved is essential in order to get people on
board and for potential projects to have a chance of success.

Initial aims will be influenced by epidemiological evidence and normative needs as well
as potential funding linked to certain issues and evidence from successful projects. It is
not feasible to consult on every aspect of community life especially within a geographical
locality, so subjects for action need to be prioritised. It is important to research the history
of interventions to avoid repeating past mistakes. Only when a full picture has been as-
similated can effective engagement within the community be planned and enacted (Public
Health England 2020; The King's Fund 2021). Workers also need to bear in mind that those
who speak the loudest or are the most active and therefore easier to reach may not be truly
representative of the community. The effort needs to be expanded in order to access less
high-profile individuals. The scope of community consultation needs to be decided upon
and this may largely depend on resources both in collecting and analysing data. Going from
house to house to ask peoples' views may reach the highest proportion of residents but are
very labour intensive. An alternative would be walking through the area at different times
of the day and chatting with local people around key issues. Conducting surveys at local
events or online surveys are other alternatives. It is important to ask about the positives as
well as the negatives as some communities can feel tarnished by a bad reputation. Once the
views of the community have been sought, the data needs to be analysed. Qualitative data
can be arranged in themes and summarised and presented with typical quotes. Quantitative
data may be presented in graphs and charts. Both will form a report with recommendations
for actions which, in turn, requires consultation. It is important that such a report be accessible to the community under focus as well as professional bodies. Therefore, it is essential
that the language is accessible and free from jargon, and it is useful to include a summary.
Dissemination needs to be planned through the local media, community groups and forums.

There are many peripheral benefits for individuals who become involved in the identification of need, action planning and project work. Participating individuals have the potential
to increase their personal skills and gain experience which can benefit both themselves and

the community in the long term. This capacity building is an essential aspect of community development work (Henderson and Thomas 2013). It is a fact that more affluent and educated communities are often more able to mobilise on issues than deprived communities due to skills already present in those communities (Murphy 2002).

A Case Study

Severe and Multiple Disadvantage – Nottingham City, UK.

This section outlines how Public Health leadership was utilised in Nottingham to promote system change and improve outcomes for individuals experiencing Severe and Multiple Disadvantage (SMD).

Severe and Multiple Disadvantage

In Nottingham, a person is considered to be experiencing SMD when they are simultaneously facing two or more of the following:

- Substance Use Issues
- Homelessness
- Offending
- Mental Health Issues
- Domestic Abuse

Literature in this field can use a variety of terms interchangeably to describe this group. Other terms commonly used are Complex Needs or Multiple Complex Needs (MCN) (McNeish et al. 2016). There is a substantial body of research highlighting the risks related to SMD, ranging from increased likelihood of facing homelessness (Fitzpatrick, Bramley and Johnsen 2013) to reduced life expectancy (Aldridge et al. 2018). There is also growing awareness that the systems designed to support individuals experiencing forms of disadvantage often work in isolation and focus on addressing one specific issue such as homelessness or mental health. This approach can fail to recognise the complex and interrelated nature of different forms of disadvantage (Fisher 2015).

Understanding Need

Nottingham is considered to have some of the highest rates of individuals experiencing SMD in England (Bramley et al. 2015). As the awareness of the needs of local residents experiencing SMD developed, the health and social care community in Nottingham focussed on understanding need and identifying barriers for the individual and the system. A health needs assessment was completed in 2019, and this provided an estimation of the number of people experiencing SMD and important insight into their needs (Everitt and Kaur 2019). This was based on extensive data and information collected through 'Opportunity Nottingham', a seven-year funded fulfilling lives programme that provided specific support for individuals with very complex needs.

This understanding was developed further through the cross-partnership working needed to support vulnerable citizens during the 'Everyone In' initiative, where, during the Covid-19 pandemic, people who were homeless or at risk of homelessness were housed in hotels in the city (House of Commons Library 2021). Nearly all of the beneficiaries of this initiative were experiencing SMD, and through this work, partners in the statutory and voluntary sector were able to come together in a way that had not been previously attempted, in order to support people sleeping rough and provide wrap-around support. This led to improved access to and engagement with a range of services.

Planning for Change

The benefits of working in this way, coupled with the knowledge that had been developed around the needs of this vulnerable cohort, were recognised by local system leaders and SMD was identified as an area of priority at the place level. The partnership that had initially been formed as a reactive response to the Covid-19 crisis grew and developed into the Nottingham City SMD Partnership. Meeting every two weeks, this partnership grew to over 100 members, taking forward areas of work to address the issues identified and also sharing knowledge and learning to promote better and more joined-up support. This partnership continued to be led by public health, but crucially it recognised and valued the expertise of all group members ranging from large agencies such as local homeless, substance use, criminal justice and mental health services to colleagues from voluntary and community sector services working with under-represented communities. Bringing together a wide variety of stakeholders, each with their own perspective on how change should be achieved, can be challenging. However, the shared focus of the partnership allowed for vital challenging conversations to take place in a positive and productive environment.

Led by public health and closely involving service users and partners, a problem-solving methodology developed by Yale University (Bradley, Nembhard and Taylor 2019) was used to develop a strategic plan to improve outcomes for people experiencing SMD. This process identified a number of key areas of focus that the partnership could take forward.

Implementing Change

In 2021, a new initiative 'Changing Futures' (Gov.uk 2021) was announced and a bid was submitted which utilised the collective knowledge of the partnership. This was successful and the partnership was awarded £4m to take forward a co-produced programme of activity to improve outcomes for people facing SMD.

Changes implemented across the system include the following:

- The development and maintenance of a multidisciplinary team that has been able to provide solutions for a number of people with very complex needs.
- The creation of a frontline service that has the right skill mix to meet the needs of the population, including the needs of women and people from our diverse communities.
- Services working in a more integrated way – for example, there are now joint working arrangements between substance misuse and mental health services.
- A support offer is now in place across key areas such as probation, primary care, mental health services, social care and housing. These specialised roles identify individuals who require additional support and then work in a joined-up way with colleagues across the system to provide workable solutions and service offers.
- Training is available to professionals across the city regarding providing effective support to those experiencing SMD.

Evaluation

The partnership has invested in research and evaluation. Evaluation includes monitoring of data around key outcomes for individuals experiencing SMD and qualitative feedback from individuals accessing services and frontline staff members attempting to provide support in this area. This process has identified that the needs of ethnically diverse communities and the needs of women are not well understood and not well reflected in the traditional definition of SMD. In response, the partnership developed two new workstreams on race equity and on gender to ensure that all work undertaken reflects the needs of the whole population.

Public Health Leadership

Attempting to achieve system change in this area has required public health leadership and input. This has included ensuring that the need is properly understood through the completion of a robust needs assessment and working in close partnership with service users and frontline workers. Public health leadership also includes utilising any strategic levers and opportunities to promote buy- in from senior leadership of key organisations. Key strategic partners must understand the work and commit to addressing the issues. In 2022, the Health and Wellbeing Board in Nottingham City identified SMD as a strategic priority, and the work of the partnership and associated progress is now reported through the city's health and wellbeing strategy's programme board. This provides visibility to the work of the partnership and also raises the issue of SMD at the senior level across the system. Work in Nottingham relating to SMD is ongoing. The aim is to sustain the progress that has been made, both for individuals and services, and to guarantee that the work continues to be a priority at a strategic level in the face of changing budgets and local priorities.

Key Messages

- Public health programmes may be primary, secondary or tertiary but health promoters tend to concentrate on primary prevention.
- Programmes are set up usually in response to policies drawn up by national and local governments and health services as a result of health needs assessment.
- Programme planning should bring together agencies and organisations and client groups who are connected with the issue in question.
- Use of a planning model is recommended and can greatly aid the planning process.
- Programmes should undertake health impact assessments of proposed initiatives to ensure programmes result in positive rather than negative outcomes for the community in question.
- Evaluation of effectiveness is a key aspect of programme planning and should be embedded from the outset.

References

Aldridge, R., Story, A., Hwang, S., Nordentoft, M., Luchenski, S., Hartwell, G. and Hayward. (2018). Morbidity and mortality in homeless individuals, prisoners, sex workers, and individuals with substance use disorders in high-income countries: A systematic review and meta-analysis. *Lancet*, 391, pp. 241–250.

American Institute for Cancer Research. (2020). *New study, a quarter of calories that children and teens eat may come from added sugars and fats* [online]. Available at: https://www.aicr.org/news/

new-study-a-quarter-of-calories-that-children-and-teens-eat-may-come-from-added-sugars-and-fats/

Asthana, S. and Halliday, J. (2006) *What works in tackling health inequalities?* Bristol: The Policy Press.

Atkins, V. (2018). *ACMD Advisory Council on the Misuse of Drugs* [online]. Available at: https://assets.publishing.service.gov.uk/government/uploads/system/uploads/attachment_data/file/761123/Vulnerability_and_Drug_Use_Report_04_Dec_.pdf

Birley, M. (2011). *Health impact assessments: Principles and practice*. Abingdon: Earthscan.

Bmj.com. (2021). *Consumption of sugar from soft drinks falls within a year of UK sugar tax | BMJ* [online]. Available at: https://www.bmj.com/company/newsroom/consumption-of-sugar-from-soft-drinks-falls-within-a-year-of-uk-sugar-tax/

Bradley, E., Nembhard, I. and Taylor, L. (2019). Leadership and management: A framework for action. In: Burns, L. and Weiner, B., eds. *Shortell & Kaluzny's health care management: Organization design and behavior*. New York: Delmar Cengage Learning, pp. 32–55.

Bramley, G., Fitzpatrick, S., Edwards, J., Ford, D., Johnsen, S., Sosenko, F. and Watkins, D. (2015). Hard edges: Mapping severe and multiple disadvantage. London: Lankelly Chase.

Centers for Disease Control and Prevention (CDC). (2013). *HIV Risk Behaviors* [online]. Available at: https://www.cdc.gov/hiv/risk/estimates/riskbehaviors.html

Davies, M. and Macdowall, W. (2006). *Health promotion theory*. Maidenhead: Open University Press.

Drug Education Forum. (2013). *Risk and protective factors*. Available at: http://www.drugeducation forum.com/index.cfm?PageID=8

Ehsan, A., Klaas, H.S., Bastianen, A. and Spini, D. (2019). Social capital and health: A systematic review of systematic reviews. *SSM - Population Health* [online], 8, p. 100425. doi: 10.1016/j.ssmph.2019.100425.

Everitt, G. and Kaur, K. (2019). *Severe multiple disadvantage (multiple needs)*. Available at: https://www.nottinghaminsight.org.uk/themes/health-and wellbeing/joint-strategic-needs-assessment/children-and-young-people/severe-multiple disadvantage-multiple-needs-2019/

Ewles, L. and Simnett, I. (2017). *Promoting health: A practical guide*. 7th ed. London: Elsevier.

Fisher, G. (2015). *The complexity of severe and multiple disadvantage*. London: Lankelly Chase.

Fitzpatrick, S., Bramley, G. and Johnsen, S. (2013). Pathways into multiple exclusion homelessness in seven UK cities. *Urban Studies*, 50(1), pp. 148–168.

Flowers, J. and Evans, S. (2020). Assessing the health of populations. In: Kawachi, I., Lang, I. and Ricciardi, W., eds. *Oxford Handbook of public health practice*. 4th ed. Oxford: Oxford University Press.

Gov.UK. (2021). *Changing futures*. Available at: https://www.gov.uk/government/collections/changing-futures

Gov.UK. (2022a). *New calorie labelling rules come into force to improve nation's health* [online]. GOV.UK. Available at: https://www.gov.uk/government/news/new-calorie-labelling-rules-come-into-force-to-improve-nations-health#:~:text=New%20legislation%20applying%20to%20large,comes%20into%20force%20on%20today.&text=New%20rules%20requiring%20calorie%20information,(Wednesday%206%20April%202022)

Gov.UK. (2022b). *Government to improve drug treatment in most deprived areas* [online]. Available at: https://www.gov.uk/government/news/government-to-improve-drug-treatment-in-most-deprived-areas

Hawtin, M. and Percy-Smith, J. (2007) *Community profiling: A practical guide*. Maidenhead, UK: Open University Press.

Henderson, P. and Thomas, N. (2013). *Skills in neighbourhood work*. 4th ed. Abingdon: Routledge.

House of Commons Library. (2021). *Coronavirus: Support for rough sleepers (England)*. Retrieved from House of Commons Library: https://commonslibrary.parliament.uk/researchbriefings/cbp-9057/

Kemm, J. (2001). Health impact assessment: A tool for healthy public policy. *Health Promotion International*, 16(1), pp. 79–85.

McCartney, G., Hearty, W., Arnot, J., Popham, F., Cumbers, A. and McMaster, R. (2019). Impact of political economy on population health: A systematic review of reviews. *American Journal of Public Health* [online], 109(6), pp. e1–e12. doi: 10.2105/ajph.2019.305001.

McNeish, D., Scott, S., Sosenko, F., Johnsen, F. and Bramley, G. (2016). *Women and girls facing severe and multiple disadvantage: An interim report*. London: Lankelly Chase.

Murphy, M. (2002). Social partnership – Is it the 'only game in town? *Community Development Journal*, 37(1), pp. 80–90.

Nice.org.uk. (2017). *Overview | Drug misuse prevention: targeted interventions | Guidance | NICE* [online]. Available at: https://www.nice.org.uk/guidance/ng64

Nuffield Council on Bioethics. (2007). *Intervention ladder*. London: Nuffield Council on Bioethics.

Nutbeam, D. (1999). The challenge to provide 'evidence' in health promotion. *Health Promotion International*, 14(2), pp. 99–101.

Nutbeam, D., Harris, E. and Wise, M. (2010). Theory in a nutshell. A practical guide to health promotion theories. Sydney, Australia: McGraw-Hill Australia Pty Ltd.

O'Connor-Fleming, M.L., Parker, E., Higgins, H. and Gould, T. (2006). A framework for evaluating health promotion program. *Health Promotion Journal of Australia*, 17(1), pp. 61–66.

Public Health England. (2018). *Introduction to evaluation in health and wellbeing* [online]. GOV.UK. Available at: https://www.gov.uk/guidance/evaluation-in-health-and-wellbeing-introduction

Public Health England. (2020). *Community-centred public health: Taking a whole system approach* [online]. GOV.UK. Available at: https://www.gov.uk/government/publications/community-centred-public-health-taking-a-whole-system-approach

Rose, G. (1992). *The strategy of preventive medicine*. Oxford: Oxford University Press.

The King's Fund. (2021). *Communities and health*. Available at: https://www.kingsfund.org.uk/publications/communities-and-health

Tolli, M.V. (2012). Effectiveness of peer education interventions for HIV prevention, adolescent pregnancy prevention and sexual health promotion for young people: A systematic review of European studies). *Health Education Research*, 27(5), pp. 904–913.

Topping, K.J. (2022). Peer education and peer counselling for health and well-being: A review of reviews. *International Journal of Environmental Research and Public Health* [online], 19(10), p. 6064. doi: 10.3390/ijerph19106064.

Villalonga-Olives, E. and Kawachi, I. (2017). The dark side of social capital: A systematic review of the negative health effects of social capital. *Social Science & Medicine* [online], 194, pp. 105–127. doi: 10.1016/j.socscimed.2017.10.020.

World Health Organization (WHO). (2001). *Evaluation in health promotion: Principles and perspectives*. Available at: http://www.euro.who.int/__data/assets/pdf_file/0007/108934/E73455.pdf

World Health Organization (WHO). (2017). *Taxes on sugary drinks: Why do it? Sugary drinks 1 – a major contributor to obesity and diabetes* [online]. Available at: http://apps.who.int/iris/bitstream/handle/10665/260253/WHO-NMH-PND-16.5Rev.1-eng.pdf

World Health Organization (WHO). (2022). *Health impact assessments* [online] Available at: https://www.who.int/tools/health-impact-assessments

9 Health Promotion for Diverse Ethnic Communities

Vanessa McFarlane

Ethnic Minorities, Demographics and Labelling

In 2019, the most common ethnic group in England and Wales remained those who classed themselves as either White British, White Irish or White other at 84.8% of the population. Indian and Black Africans were the second and third largest populations, respectively (Office for National Statistics 2020). As populations of countries become more and more diverse, countries seeking to assess the needs of various communities and construct services to meet these needs have struggled with the semantics of labelling. In the UK, various terms have been used over time to describe the non-indigenous population. Terms like Black and Minority Ethnic (BME) divided these populations into just two categories, those considered as 'black' and others considered not 'black'. Much of the UK's non-white population moved to the UK as a result of the 1948 British Nationality Act (Legislation.gov.uk 2022) which gave former British colonial subjects mainly from the Indian subcontinent, Africa and the Caribbean right to settle in the UK. More recently, we have seen the use of Black Asian Minority Ethnic (BAME) to 'lump' together anyone who is not from the white community. More recently, EU migrants and asylum seekers have increased the diversity of the population making such broad categories a nonsense. Unfortunately, this coalescing together of disparate groups can hide the realities of inequalities within these groupings and may produce statistics which being an average of the whole does a disservice to certain minorities within them. As a consequence, statistics on diversity can look better than they are. The NHS Race and Health Observatory (2022) states that 'the "BAME" category has lost virtually all analytical values. Put simply, a BAME person simply does not exist'. This has obvious consequences for health needs assessment and tailored service provision. London continues to be the most ethnically diverse city in the UK with less than half the population at 48.4% identifying as White British compared to 78.8% for England and Wales overall. The way groups identify themselves may differ over time, possibly as a result of greater integration. Some children of ethnic minority backgrounds in the UK are now fourth generation born in this country, whereas others will have been born in another country. Both the increase in diverse populations and greater integration have significant challenges for the provision of health services which have to be flexible, innovative and fair in the way they deal with communities in order to improve their health. Language and terms to describe the UK's growing and changing ethnic minority population have to continually evolve with the population. It will be very difficult to find an all-encompassing term to represent all the groups that are not the majority. Maybe if we are able to achieve a fairer society where inequalities are no longer so stark, then the need for these labels will become less relevant. This chapter will refer to ethnic minority communities or people from ethnic minority backgrounds and will

DOI: 10.4324/9781003411321-9

include white minorities (such as Gypsy, Roma or Travellers and other white minorities) in line with Government guidance (GOV.UK 2022).

Racism

Racism and discrimination continue to have an impact on the lives of ethnic minority communities living in the UK. Recently this has been brought to the mainstream public attention by the growth of the Black Lives Matter protest movement and the Windrush Scandal. The latter came about in 2018 when early Caribbean settlers to the UK who were invited into the country as a result of the 1948 Act to plug the workforce gap and at the time were not required to have passport documentation were challenged by the UK Home Office as to their right to remain. This resulted in many people being wrongly deported and children of these migrants without proof of citizenship were left without access to benefits, healthcare, social care and housing. This scandal is an example of 'othering', which refers to the conscious or unconscious assumption that a group poses a threat to the favoured group. This can be based on any aspect that may be different about that person, language, religion, sexual identity, etc. It usually creates processes of exclusion and dehumanisation (Very Well Mind 2022). Intersectionality is another useful term and refers to multiple factors of advantage or disadvantage a person may experience. Being a white, heterosexual male would put an individual in a position of advantage when you consider how society is structured. Whereas a woman of Indian heritage, who identified as lesbian, would experience three aspects of her identity that could put her at a disadvantage in society. These overlapping social identities can be empowering or oppressive. Intersectionality has its roots in the feminist movement when it was identified that women have different experiences of discrimination depending on their social identity. The feminist movement was predominantly white and middle class which is not representative of all women, particularly those from an ethnic minority background. Attitudes to asylum seekers are another prime example of 'othering', but despite the public backlash, refugees and asylum seekers only make up 1% of the UK population (UNHCR 2013).

Health Inequalities Based on Ethnicity

Following on from the introduction to health inequalities in Chapter 3, this chapter will explore the issue of how ethnicity impacts the health of ethnic minority people living in the UK. Differences in health status can be experienced by different factors such as an individual's minority background, socio-economic status, geographical location, disability and sex. The way these factors 'intersect' can influence the health inequalities an individual experiences (The King's Fund 2022). There is a plethora of research over the years focussing on the health inequalities experienced by people from ethnic minority backgrounds. In 2022, the NHS Race and Health Observatory identified 178 studies highlighting widespread ethnic inequalities in the areas they reviewed. The key contributing factors stated were as follows:

- Structural, institutional and interpersonal racism
- Lack of appropriate treatment for health conditions
- Poor quality or discriminatory treatment by healthcare staff
- Lack of high-quality ethnic monitoring data recorded by the NHS
- Lack of appropriate interpreting service
- Delays in or avoiding seeking help for health problems due to fear of racist treatment
(NHS Race and Health Observatory 2022)

We again though need to recognise the differences within ethnic minority communities; for example, both the Pakistani and Bangladeshi groups reported more limiting long-term illness and poorer health than the White British group, but the White Gypsy and Irish Traveller groups reported poorest health (The King's Fund 2021). Economic migrants to the UK tend to be young and so are more likely to be in good health, so the disadvantage in knowledge of and access to healthcare and the inequalities that they face may only become apparent later in life (Migration Observatory 2021).

The NHS Constitution establishes the principles and values of the NHS in England. Some of these principles are clearly based on equality in particular:

- The NHS provides a comprehensive service, available to all.
- Access to NHS services is based on clinical need, not the individual's ability to pay.
- The patient will be at the heart of everything the NHS does.

These are important values, but unfortunately for people from ethnic minority backgrounds, it is not their lived experience. Research has shown that services are not available to all in the same way. This will be examined in more detail later. Refugees and asylum seekers are often questioned about their status when accessing services, in some cases being wrongly billed for healthcare provision. This has impacted those particular groups, making them avoid healthcare services for fear it will impact their immigration status. This is not putting the individual at the heart of everything the NHS does.

The following section will focus on key health issues for ethnic minority communities.

Mental Health

In 2017 the UK Government commissioned a review of its 1983 Mental Health Act. The author of the subsequent report, Professor Simon Wessley, openly points to ongoing unconscious bias and structural and institutional racism as contributors to the ongoing inequalities experienced by ethnic minority groups. There is evidence to show that the experience of racism and the fear of experiencing racism and racist attacks impact the mental health of people from minority groups. It contributes to chronic stress and also affects children due to the worsening mental health of their parents (GOV.UK 2017). We can see intersectionality of circumstances or characteristics in play here (genetics, childhood experiences, adult environment and experiences) that also mean those from ethnic minority backgrounds are more vulnerable to experiencing mental ill health (GOV. UK 2017).

The NHS Race and Health Observatory Report (2022) carried out a literature review on ethnic inequalities in mental health services with a focus on the past 10 years. Recurring themes are as follows:

- Lack of trust in healthcare professionals which delays seeking help. This showed up in a lack of trust in those in authority such as family doctors. People felt that their experiences of racism and discrimination were not understood and that models of recovery did not take into account these experiences.
- Difficulty in navigating healthcare systems.
- Language barriers and the lack of good quality interpreting services. How can you explain how you feel if someone cannot understand what you are saying?

The barriers experienced by the adult population were similar for young people from ethnic minority backgrounds with young people also having a fear of being held in mental services, being given medication and not being released. Two large studies found that Black children were 10 times more likely to be referred to CAMHS via social services in comparison to White British children (NHS Race and Health Observatory 2022).

Access rates for Improving Access to Psychological Therapy (IAPT) or talking therapies were lower for all ethnic groups compared to White British people and referrals generally came from secondary care or community services rather than from family doctors or self-referral (NHS Race and Health Observatory 2022). There has also long been the issue of culturally appropriate therapy when the world of therapy is predominantly white. As mentioned earlier, people of ethnic minority backgrounds often feel their healthcare providers do not have an understanding of their experiences, particularly racism which often contributes to their mental ill health. To go to therapy and sit in front of someone you don't feel will understand you can negate the whole purpose of the therapy.

Other studies have found that Black and Mixed White and Black groups reported greater levels of unfair treatment from mental health services and staff (NHS Race and Health Observatory 2022). This persistent lack of trust in mental health services which comes from negative experiences felt by people of ethnic minority backgrounds leads to delays in accessing treatment which means the individuals may end up in crisis situations that may involve the police and be referred to services via this route, which is much more negative and traumatic.

Maternal Healthcare

Better collection of ethnic data has revealed persistent ethnic inequalities in maternal, perinatal and infant health which has shown an elevated risk of maternal mortality amongst Black and Asian women when compared to White women (NHS Race and Health Observatory 2022). Poor outcomes are also high for women living in the most deprived areas of the country. This brings in the issue of intersectionality for women from ethnic minority backgrounds if they are already living in deprivation they are at a double disadvantage.

There have been initiatives to focus on improving equity for 'all' mothers and babies. The MBRRACE-UK's Saving Lives, Improving Mothers' Care report (2021) stated that Black women are four times more likely to die in pregnancy and childbirth, with mixed ethnicity and Asian women two times more likely. Maternal deaths are relatively rare in the western world, but disparities are very serious and need to be highlighted. A number of studies into the experiences of ethnic minority women have revealed issues that affect women's perception of maternal services and the treatment they receive which can impact how they engage with these services. The ability of the healthcare providers to engender trust and provide essential information and test for understanding was an important theme in helping women maintain contact with services. Some women felt that their accents impacted how they were viewed, with professionals assuming they lacked understanding or education. Language continues to be a huge barrier, with the lack of information in different languages and the lack of quality interpreting services continuing to be reported as an issue. Higginbottom and colleagues (2020) found that for Somali women, language was the main factor undermining communication with health providers. Watson and Downe (2017) also found this with Romani women. When English is a second language and communication is poor, women felt unsafe and vulnerable and felt that their needs were not being met. This can be another layer of intersectionality experienced by migrant women and refugee and asylum seeking women.

Women who have had negative experiences with maternal services in the past found it difficult to form positive relationships in subsequent pregnancies (Khan 2021) and some groups such as Travellers may prefer to rely on their own communities rather than engage with healthcare services (McFadden, Siebelt and Gavine 2018). More understanding of cultural norms and how communities support pregnant women is needed to ensure women from ethnic minority backgrounds get the care they need at the time they need it.

In 2022, a new charity FIVEXMORE produced the 'Black Maternity Experience Report' that presents the testimony of over 1300 Black and Black Mixed Race women. They report that Black women are twice as likely to have severe pregnancy complications or near misses and these are much more frequent. The report highlighted three key areas of concern with regard to healthcare staff:

- Attitudes – including racist and dismissive behaviour
- Knowledge – this included a lack of knowledge regarding Black women's anatomy and physiology
- Assumptions – often around pain tolerance of Black women being higher, their education being lower and their relationship status

These recurring themes come up in a number of reports and research and contribute to ethnic minority women feeling 'othered'. Research regularly highlights systemic and institutional racism as a significant contributor to the care of pregnant women. This is not to say that White women do not face poor attitudes and stereotyping by healthcare staff, but the additional issue of racism and discrimination has an additional impact on women from ethnic minority backgrounds (NHS Race and Health Observatory 2022). For asylum seeking women, there are the additional difficulties around immigration issues, navigating an unfamiliar healthcare services and discriminatory treatment from staff resulting in isolation, late presentation and feeling unsafe or threatened.

The FIVEXMORE report does highlight the positive experiences Black women have had within maternity services and this was due to cultural awareness of staff, mixed ethnicity staff teams, and healthcare staff having a patient centred approach and women having the opportunity to discuss culturally sensitive issues such as female genital mutilation.

Sexual Health

In 2019, statistics from the US Sexual Transmitted Infections (STIs) Surveillance showed that people from ethnic minority backgrounds are disproportionately affected by STIs (CDC 2021). In the UK, the rate of gonorrhoea in ethnic communities is 3.5 times higher and for trichomoniasis it is nine times higher than it is for the general population (HIV Prevention England 2022). In 2021, Public Health England produced its 'STIs: promoting the sexual health and wellbeing of people from a Black Caribbean Background' report in an attempt to address sexual health inequalities in this community. As a result, the Department of Health and Social Care (DHSC) set out the following goals:

- To reverse the rapid increase in STIs in populations most at risk of infections
- To use its data, evidence, evaluations, etc. to undertake activities to reduce STIs and promote safer sexual behaviours

It is important to point out that although STI rates are higher amongst people of Black ethnicity, this varies. Black African ethnicities have relatively lower rates of common STIs, although they have greater HIV rates. Black Africans make up less than 2% of the UK population, but one in six people who are newly diagnosed with HIV are Black African and 29% of people living with HIV are Black African (Tht.org.uk 2020). Contributing factors for the rates of HIV in these populations are that although people come from countries where there are high rates of HIV, they often don't know they are positive until they get to the UK and get tested. Some women have been victims of rape in their home countries and have contracted HIV as a result. Some people are fearful of anything affecting their immigration status and so are reluctant to be tested, thinking that this will be a barrier to their emigration. The major issue for the Black African community is late presentation, which in the case of HIV is detrimental as a delay in diagnosis may mean that the virus has already started to attack the immune system (Tht.org.uk 2020).

Public Health England (2021) conducted research which suggests that Black Caribbean men tend to have first sex at an earlier age, have more sexual partners and are less monogamous than White men. However, there was no discernible difference in the sexual behaviour of Black Caribbean women compared to White women. Nevertheless, issues such as the intersection of ethnicity and gender, how women's experiences of coercion and violence related to their risk of STIs and unplanned pregnancies, together with issues of power imbalances in negotiating safer sex associated with how women are perceived as sexual objects, all have an impact on their sexual health.

Young people are still most likely to be diagnosed with an STI. A small study of 71 young people aged 17 to 25 was carried out in Brighton and Hove (Health Watch and Young Healthwatch 2019); the young people had good knowledge of the sexual health services and had a good experience using them. They also had good access to sexual health information via school. However, the barriers for some young people in this research were as follows:

- Language – for those new to the UK and when English is a second language
- Confidentiality – fears that services might share information with parents
- Culture/religious factors – issues around sex being taboo, consequences of parents knowing they were sexually active, being scared to be seen at the clinic and not accessing services due to feeling of guilt or fear of being judged

Some of these issues were a major barrier for young people from Asian and African backgrounds where cultural and religious restrictions may be felt more. This could be the same for refugee and asylum seeking young people who may be coming from countries where sex is taboo and is compounded by their lack of knowledge of UK healthcare systems.

Ways Forward

Unfortunately, despite the persistence of health inequalities, the last ten years has seen effective health promotion initiatives and ethnic health projects being either discontinued or merged into mainstream services. Research into priorities and potential solutions and recommendations are manifest; there needs to be:

- Improvements in provision for those where English is a second language, both written material and good quality interpreters to remove the persistent language barrier that is generational.
- Training for staff to be more culturally sensitive and appropriate and to promote anti-racist practices as racism continues to be a major contributor to health inequalities for people from ethnic minority backgrounds who have felt excluded, discriminated against

and treated less well by healthcare professionals. Training needs to be ongoing rather than a one-off tokenistic event that has little impact.

- More involvement and co creation with ethnic minority communities when it comes to services, listening and acting on the many pieces of qualitative research that have taken place over the years and implementing change based on what has been shared.
- Improvements in ethnic data collection. The way data is collected is not robust and the ethnic categories are too simplified and not representative of the huge diversity that exists. Currently some services will collect systematic ethnic data which is then used to identify further research gaps, needs and patterns. Other services may collect ethnic data only as a tickbox activity. There needs to be more consistency in ethnic monitoring.

We need to move away from the erroneous perception that because many ethnic communities are third or fourth generation and born in the country in which they now live that assimilation has removed the need for specialist services. Pervasive racism and economic and health inequalities persist for a substantial proportion of the minority ethnic population and need to be addressed.

Critical Thinking

Considering the factors contributing to poorer health and healthcare for people from an ethnic minority background,

Why do you think these inequalities have not been tackled properly?
Is the NHS living up to its constitution and abiding by the Equality Act 2010?
What will happen if we continue on this path?
What do you think are the key strategies for redressing the balance?

Key Messages

- Inequalities based on ethnicity have improved little over the decades.
- Research has confirmed that racism and discrimination continue to be a huge contributing factor to the quality of healthcare given to people of ethnic minority backgrounds.
- There needs to be a systemic change to address these inequalities which will require a financial commitment.

References

CDC. (2021). *Sexually transmitted disease surveillance, 2019* [online]. Centers for Disease Control and Prevention. Available at: https://www.cdc.gov/std/statistics/2019/default.htm
FIVEXMORE. (2022). *Black maternity experience report*. Available at: https://www.fivexmore.com/blackmereport
GOV.UK. (2017). *Independent Review of the Mental Health Act* [online]. Available at: https://www.gov.uk/government/groups/independent-review-of-the-mental-health-act
GOV.UK. (2022). Writing about ethnicity - GOV.UK. Available at: ethnicity-facts-figures.service.gov.uk
Health Watch and Young Healthwatch. (2019). *Exploring the views and experiences of young people from BAME (Black, Asian, and minority ethnic groups) backgrounds around local sexual health*

services. Available at Young-Healthwatch-BAME-Sexual-Health-report-April-2020.pdf (health watchbrightonandhove.co.uk)

Higginbottom, G.M., Evans, C., Morgan, M., Bharj, K.K., Eldridge, J., Hussain, B. and Salt, K. (2020). *Access to and interventions to improve maternity care services for immigrant women: A narrative synthesis systematic review.* Available at: https://pubmed.ncbi.nlm.nih.gov/32207887/

HIV Prevention England. (2022). *HIV Prevention England* [online]. Available at: https://www. hivpreventionengland.org.uk/

Khan, Z. (2021). Ethnic health inequalities in the UK's maternity services: A systematic literature review. *British Journal of Midwifery*, 29(2), pp. 100–107. doi: 10.12968/bjom.2021.29.2.100.

Legislation.gov.uk. (2022). *British Nationality Act 1948* [online]. Available at: https://www.legislation. gov.uk/ukpga/Geo6/11-12/56/enacted

MBRRACE-UK. (2021). *Saving lives, improving mothers' care report.* Available at: https://www. birthcompanions.org.uk/resources/mbrrace-uk-saving-lives-improving-mothers-care-2021

McFadden, A., Siebelt, L. and Gavine, A. (2018). Gypsy, Roma and Traveller access to and engagement with health services: A systematic review. *European Journal of Public Health*, 28(1), pp. 74–81. doi: 10.1093/eurpub/ckx226.

Migration Observatory. (2021). *The health of migrants in the UK - Migration Observatory* [online]. Available at: https://migrationobservatory.ox.ac.uk/resources/briefings/the-health-of-migrants-in-the-uk/

NHS Race and Health Observatory. (2022). *Ethnic inequalities in healthcare: A rapid evidence review - NHS Race and Health Observatory* [online]. Available at: https://www.nhsrho.org/ publications/ethnic-inequalities-in-healthcare-a-rapid-evidence-review/

Office for National Statistics (ONS). (2020). *Population estimates for the UK, England and Wales, Scotland and Northern Ireland* [online]. Ons.gov.uk. Available at: https://www.ons.gov. uk/peoplepopulationandcommunity/populationandmigration/populationestimates/bulletins/ annualmidyearpopulationestimates/mid2019estimates

Public Health England. (2021). Sexually transmitted infections: Promoting the sexual health and wellbeing of people from a Black Caribbean background. Available at: https://www.gov.uk/government/ publications/promoting-the-sexual-health-and-wellbeing-of-people-from-a-black-caribbean-background-an-evidence-based-resource

The King's Fund. (2021). The health of people from ethnic minority groups in England | The King's Fund. Available at: https://www.kingsfund.org.uk/publications/health-people-ethnic-minority-groups-england

The King's Fund. (2022). *What are health inequalities?* [online]. Available at: https://www.kingsfund. org.uk/publications/what-are-health-inequalities

Tht.org.uk. (2020). *Newly diagnosed | Terrence Higgins Trust* [online]. Available at: https://www. tht.org.uk/hiv-and-sexual-health/being-diagnosed-hiv/newly-diagnosed#:~:text=Late%20diagnosis% 20means%20that%20you,is%20considered%20a%20late%20diagnosis

UNHCR. (2013). *UNHCR Global Trends 2013* [online]. Available at: https://www.unhcr.org/uk/ statistics/country/5399a14f9/unhcr-global-trends-2013.html

Very Well Mind. (2022). *What is othering?* Available at: verywellmind.com

Watson, H.L. and Downe, S. (2017). Discrimination against childbearing Romani women in maternity care in Europe: A mixed-methods systematic review. *Reproductive Health* [online], 14(1). doi: 10.1186/s12978-016-0263-4.

10 Mental Health Promotion, Psychological Therapies and Young People's Mental Health

Matthew Horrocks

Introduction

The mental health and well-being of young people is a key consideration for modern societies, and this chapter will focus on mental health promotion for young people. In particular, this chapter will explore the application of cognitive behavioural psychological therapies to promote good mental health and well-being.

The Mental Health of Young People

Young people as a group are often defined as encompassing the United Nations (UN) and World Health Organization's definitions of children (0–9 years old), adolescents (10–19 years old) and youths (15–24 years old).

Childhood is characterised by key developmental and emotional milestones where children learn healthy life skills and how to cope in the event of problems (Centre for Disease Control and Prevention 2022). Adolescence is characterised as a critical formative time, for developing social and emotional habits, where young people experience emotional and social changes which can fundamentally shape their mental health (World Health Organization 2021). Youth is best understood as a period of transition from the dependence of childhood to adulthood and independence, including leaving compulsory education and seeking paid employment (United Nations 2013).

Global bodies such as the United Nations recognise that across the world the lives of young people can be affected by poverty, poor nutrition, variable access to healthcare and education, occurrence of violence and conflict and higher rates of unemployment compared with adults (United Nations 2022a, 2022b).

Against this backdrop of dynamic structural, regional, societal, economic and cultural factors, young people's mental health is a high priority for health and social care systems across the world.

It is estimated that globally, 13% of adolescents live with a diagnosed mental disorder (United Nations Children's Fund 2021) and one in seven aged 10–19 experiences a mental disorder, many of which are neither recognised nor appropriately treated (World Health Organization 2021). Common mental health problems amongst young people can include anxiety, depression, eating disorders, psychosis and neurodevelopmental disorders, such as attention deficit hyperactivity disorder (ADHD). The impact of such mental health problems on young people can include reduced attendance or participation in education, social or emotional withdrawal, increased risk-taking in relation to alcohol, substance use or sexual behaviours and increased chances of being involved in interpersonal violence, self-harm or death by suicide (World Health Organization 2021).

DOI: 10.4324/9781003411321-10

The Covid-19 pandemic was associated with increased levels of mental health distress across many population groups globally, including young people. Symptoms reported included those associated with anxiety and depression, sleep disturbance and psychological trauma reactions (Dragioti et al. 2022). A recent meta-analysis reported that the prevalence of anxiety and depression amongst young people doubled during the pandemic and was worse in older adolescents and girls (Racine et al. 2021). Another pooled analysis of cohort studies suggests that the deterioration in mental health triggered by living through the pandemic might be sustained over time and maintained by increased financial stress and disruptions to daily life and social relationships (Patel et al. 2022). Conversely, other studies have suggested that different mental health trajectories were observable amongst the population as a result of the pandemic, including improvement and stability as well as deterioration (Shevlin et al. 2021). The long-term impact of the pandemic on mental health is still being observed, but it is considered likely that the effects of the pandemic on global mental health will continue to be experienced for years to come (United Nations 2020).

Concerningly, even prior to the pandemic, some studies suggested psychological distress appeared to be rising amongst young people in westernised economies, with increasing rates of depression and anxiety reported (Thapar et al. 2022; Twenge et al. 2019). Critics have argued that rather than actual increases in prevalence, the increases in reported symptoms may reflect overall increases in population size, greater public awareness of mental health issues and improved screening, diagnosis and access to treatment (Baxter et al. 2014).

Despite the contested claims as to whether distress in young people is actually increasing, there is no doubt that mental health remains a key consideration for the well-being of young people. In England, 50% of mental health problems are estimated to have onset by age 14, and 75% of lifelong mental health conditions are estimated to have started by the age of 24 (Royal College of Paediatrics and Child Health 2020).

Research data suggests that recent years have seen a large increase in the number of young people seeking help for mental health distress, particularly in regard to anxiety disorders, depression, self-harm, eating disorders, autistic spectrum disorders and ADHD (Cybulski et al. 2021). Correspondingly, a substantial increase in the number of primary healthcare family doctor consultations with young people relating to anxiety or depressive symptoms has been recorded (Slee et al. 2021).

This rising demand for mental health support is occurring in a context where many NHS staff report high levels of stress, exhaustion and burnout stemming from the impacts of the Covid-19 pandemic (Liberati et al. 2021; Newman, Jeve and Majumder 2022). These post-pandemic consequences are exacerbating longer term problems in the NHS, where staff are facing unprecedentedly high workloads, high stress levels and a fear of persecution amidst a climate of fear and bullying to achieve targets (Wilkinson 2015). Meanwhile, NHS provider organisations are struggling with significant financial strain, large numbers of unfilled posts and a demand for care which is outstripping capacity (Appleby 2019; NHS providers 2017; Palmer and Rolewicz 2022). This has produced a dual problem of both increased demand and reduced resources. Despite incredible efforts from their staff, NHS mental health providers are experiencing increasing pressures resulting in high waiting times (Plewes 2022), leading to a mental health system described as overburdened, underfunded and failing to prevent avoidable distress (Bannister 2021).

In this context, the need for healthcare systems to re-engage with public health approaches in mental health is vital. Such an approach offers a way to respond to the surge in demand, reduced treatment capacity and the ongoing societal conditions which may contribute to increasing mental health distress. An urgent and proactive re-engagement with concepts of early intervention and mental health promotion appears essential.

Defining Mental Health Promotion

Mental health promotion (MHP) has been defined as 'aiming to promote positive mental health, by increasing psychological well-being, competence and resilience, by creating supporting living conditions and environments' (World Health Organization 2004, p. 17). This definition might seem a bit broad, and a bit abstract, so let's try to explore some of the concepts which it raises. It is important to note that the terms used in the World Health Organization's report can have different meanings in the wider literature, and so a selective overview is presented here.

Psychological well-being has been defined as more than the absence of ill-being, but also encompassing the combination of feeling good, functioning effectively and having the sense that life is going well (Huppert 2009). Such a definition does not claim that psychological well-being precludes people from experiencing difficult situations or painful emotions, which are a normal part of life. Instead, this definition suggests that to be in a state of well-being, a person should not be experiencing ongoing enduring emotional pain or having to tolerate circumstances which interfere with their ability to function in their daily life.

Psychological competence has been defined as an individual being able to meet the developmental tasks expected of them, at a given age and in particular cultural and historical contexts. Such developmental tasks can include deploying appropriate emotional regulation strategies and appropriately managing interpersonal interaction (O'Connor et al. 2022).

Resilience has been described as the process and outcome of successfully adapting to difficult or challenging life experiences through the use of a repertoire of flexible mental, emotional and behavioural adjustments to internal and external demands (American Psychological Association 2022). Scholars in this field of research highlight that resilience is a dynamic, rather than static, quality, which can fluctuate across the lifespan, and across situations, contexts and levels of adversity (Denckla et al. 2020).

These three concepts (well-being, competence and resilience) suggest that good mental health is partly an individual concern, partly an interpersonal outcome and partly a consequence of social, environmental and contextual circumstances. It has long been regarded that mental health is shaped by an individual's biology, their psychological responses and social context or social conditions. This combination was described in the 1970s as the 'biopsychosocial' model of mental health (Engel 1977). However, the current definitions of well-being, competence and resilience provide nuance to the biopsychosocial model by highlighting that mental health is a fluctuating state in which the social context and circumstance play a very significant mediating role.

The WHO's 2004 definition of MHP draws attention to the inseparable link between living conditions and environmental conditions as facilitating or preventing well-being, competence and resilience. In recent work, the WHO has stated that MHP involves activities intended to identify individual, social and structural determinants of mental health, and then intervening to reduce risks, build resilience and establish supportive environments for mental health (World Health Organization 2022).

The term structural determinants of mental health refers to how people's mental health is shaped by the circumstances in which they are born, grow, live, work and age, and the impact of societal inequality whereby people with lower social status have been repeatedly shown to be at higher risk of poor mental health (Alegría et al. 2018). Inequalities which act as structural determinants of mental health can include the unequal distribution of power, money and resources across society (World Health Organization and Calouste Gulbenkian Foundation 2014). Other structural determinants may include racism, sexism, violence, discrimination or other unfavourable social, economic or environmental circumstances giving rise to inequality (Compton and Shim 2015). Evidence shows that across the UK there is a clear relationship between social inequalities and worsening physical and mental health and mortality (Marmot et al. 2010). Moreover, it has been shown in a cross national analysis that people living in societies where wealth is more equally distributed are less likely to experience mental ill health (Wilkinson and Pickett 2009). However, within the UK contemporary data suggests that social inequalities, such as the gap between rich and poor, are increasing (Marmot et al. 2020). A consequence of this widening social inequality is that in poorer areas people have a reduction in life expectancy and worse ill health, along with greater levels of child poverty, less educational attainment, greater risk of exclusion from school and greater risk of youth crime (Marmot et al. 2020). Therefore, acknowledgement of the widening social inequality in the UK and the increasingly visible impacts of structural determinants of poor health are unavoidable considerations in contemporary understandings of mental health and MHP.

The promotion of good mental health, therefore, needs to account for social and structural determinants. Such a view is fundamental to public health, since mental health is, in turn, a determinant of physical health and well-being. However, MHP has been relatively neglected within the public health sphere (Faculty of Public Health and Mental Health Foundation 2016). Traditionally, a distinction has been made in public mental health between the concepts of Universal, Selective and Indicated approaches (Institute of Medicine Committee on Prevention of Mental Disorders 1994). Based on earlier work, the Institute of Medicine Committee on Prevention of Mental Disorders (1994) described these concepts as follows:

- Universal approaches are those which should apply to *everybody* in a specific population to prevent ill health.
- Selective approaches are those which are indicated when *a subgroup* of the population is at a higher than average risk, even though some members of the subgroup may not go on to manifest the condition or concern.
- Indicated approaches are those which apply when *an individual* has been identified as being at higher risk.

Historically, these definitions might be understood as the prevention and treatment of mental health problems. However, MHP has been differentiated from the concepts of 'treatment' and 'prevention' of mental disorders, although these can be seen as related but different activities (World Health Organization 2004). Mental health treatment could be described as a course of action, including diagnosis, application of treatment methods, and evaluation of progress or prognosis, in a deliberate and intentional way to alleviate distress or pathological symptoms. In contrast, prevention of mental health distress has been defined as specific attempts to prevent or reduce the risk of mental health distress from occurring (Institute of Medicine Committee on Prevention of Mental Disorders 1994). It has been argued that the boundary between prevention and treatment can be hard to distinguish, for example, in the case of psychosocial interventions such as educational programmes (Purgato et al. 2020). However, MHP, as we have seen, is about working with individuals and communities, in a way which encompasses treatment and prevention, but also extends towards attempts to strengthen positive aspects of mental health and enhance well-being and qualities of life (Kobau et al. 2011). It has been argued that to account for these issues, practitioners need to shift their gaze from individual patients towards recognising how societal institutions, policies, and conditions influence the mental health of individuals (Bailey 2020). Since social and structural determinants of mental health transcend different fields of clinical specialisation and across academic subject areas, MHP can be seen as a multidisciplinary area of practice which aims to enhance well-being and quality of life for individuals, communities and society in general (Jané-Llopis et al. 2005).

Potential Interventions to Improve the Mental Health of Young People

Given the large range of known causes of poor mental health and the wide scope of MHP in seeking to promote better well-being across society, potential MHP interventions are, therefore, multifaceted and likely to include structural, societal and individual interventions.

Structural interventions are attempts to restructure society to create more equal opportunities and to reduce social inequality. Examples of structural interventions can include public health policies and programmes to increase nutrition, financial assistance, and access to educational and healthcare provision.

Societal interventions can include attempts to create communities and living conditions which are more likely to build positive mental health and well-being. Examples of such interventions could include home visiting or early intervention, parenting training programmes, pre-school and school based programmes, the provision of adequate housing, and interventions which seek to build and strengthen community capacity and well-being.

Individual approaches can include specific programmes aimed at developing personal skills, resilience and social competence, or targeted support, such as a brief psychological intervention in primary care following a major life event. For individuals, one of the most effective interventions is cognitive behavioural therapy (CBT), which will be described in the next section.

Further Reading

For an excellent overview of a range of evidence-based structural, societal and individual MHP interventions, see the review paper by Jané-Llopis et al. (2005).

Cognitive Behavioural Therapies (CBT)

CBT is not a singular decontextualised intervention; instead, CBT is an umbrella term describing a range of related therapies, which are empirically grounded in the importance of clinical science and the clinical application of specific interventions (Stott et al. 2010). Empirically grounded interventions are those deriving from a clear theoretical basis, featuring a strong grasp of the phenomenology and epidemiology of clinical problems, and applying treatment approaches tested in ecologically valid experimental studies and randomised controlled trials evaluating outcomes at the population level (Salkovskis 2002).

Within the umbrella term of CBT, there are distinct approaches which emphasise behavioural or cognitive interventions. These approaches include cognitive therapy, behavioural therapy, schema focused therapy, mindfulness-based cognitive therapy, acceptance and commitment therapy, dialectical behaviour therapy and rational emotive behavioural therapy (McMain et al. 2015). Cumulatively therefore,, CBT is the most researched form of psychological therapy, with no other psychological therapy consistently outperforming CBT, leading to CBT being described as the gold standard of psychological intervention (David, Cristea and Hofmann 2018). David, Cristea and Hofmann (2018) go on to argue that CBT approaches are such effective interventions because they are empirically grounded, target defined psychopathologies with specific treatment strategies and are underpinned by decades of research into information processing and the role of cognitions in mediating emotions and behaviours. Whilst CBT places an important emphasis on exploring situational cognition, CBT is actually also all about understanding, exploring and managing emotional and behavioural reactions. Cognitions and cognitive processes are emphasised because they can provide direct pathways to relevant emotions and behaviours which can help people to explore their reactions and manage their psychological and emotional well-being.

Activity

Write out or talk out loud your reaction to this scenario.
   Imagine you are asleep in bed at night but wake up hearing the sound of something smashing in the kitchen downstairs.

- What thought goes through your mind as you awoke?
- What emotions are triggered in you?
- What would you notice in your body at that time?
- What would you do?

Next, explore this scenario:
   As you wake up, you remember that you have a pet cat that likes to jump onto the kitchen counter and you had a glass of milk before bed, but you left the glass on the kitchen counter.

- Are your thoughts, emotions, bodily reactions and behaviours the same or different?

Are there differences if you attribute the sound to your cat rather than a more sinister cause such as a burglar? That's not to say that you might not still need to go downstairs and take some action, but you might experience the situation differently.
   This is the essence of CBT approaches: exploring how you think, your appraisal of the situation, how you react and whether your reactions are justified and helpful in context and whether they are promoting or detracting from your sense of well-being.

CBT often focuses on how aspects of an individual's experience are triggered in a present-day situation, but CBT also explores how people develop psychological problems and how further problems might be prevented (Wills and Sanders 2013). Understanding the reciprocal links between cognitions (thoughts) and cognitive processes, emotions, behavioural responses and physiological reactions as components of experiencing and reacting can help people to generate and test out potential other ways of responding. Specific applications of CBT approaches to promote better mental health by helping people to manage their emotions, thoughts and behaviours are outlined below.

Managing Unhelpful Automatic Thoughts

In early CBT research, Aaron Beck (1963) noticed negative biases in the way that people experiencing psychological distress thought. People prone to depression typically reported thoughts characterised by self-blame, self-criticism and a sense of being overwhelmed, whereas people prone to anxiety reported a sense of danger or threat and wanting to escape (Beck 1963). In later work, Beck suggested the concept of 'automatic thoughts' where people prone to psychological distress would experience frequent, spontaneous and seemingly plausible intrusive thoughts which served to maintain and intensify psychological distress (Beck 1976). Subsequent clinical practice and research have confirmed that people struggling with mental health problems are much more likely to think in ways that are biased or distorted, which sustains and prolongs mental health distress. Beck called these changes in ways of thinking 'biased processing of information' because a person with mental health distress often has a tendency to think in biased ways that extend or prolong their problems (Beck 1997). Beck's theory suggested that one's feelings are shaped, to a very large extent, by the way one interprets experience. CBT recognises that the relationship between emotion and cognition is bidirectional and reciprocal, yet the way we perceive events or situations strongly influences our emotions (Hofmann, Asmundson and Beck 2013). Therefore, cognition is strongly linked to our regulation of emotion and behaviour, so learning to manage automatic thoughts is a key skill in CBT.

Promoting Psychological Flexibility

Increasing psychological flexibility, or being able to take a step back from thoughts and ensuing responses, by noticing and being curious about these reactions is an important skill that CBT helps people to develop. This skill is sometimes called 'decentering' or the ability to notice inner events, without excessively and unconstructively reacting to those inner experiences (Bennett et al. 2021). This process has been described as shifting focus from within one's subjective experience onto that experience (Bernstein et al. 2015). Being able to shift focus this way helps individuals manage stressors and build alternative ways of responding, which are particularly effective when informed by deeply held personal values (Gloster, Meyer and Lieb 2017). Developing psychological flexibility has been described as fundamental to good health, particularly in the context of stressors and other socioenvironmental factors which detract from psychological well-being (Kashdan and Rottenberg 2010). CBT approaches can help people to increase their psychological flexibility and, by association, improve their quality of life and enhance psychological well-being (Lucas and Moore 2019).

Emotional Regulation

Emotional regulation has been defined as the process by which individuals influence the emotions they have, and when and how they experience them (Gross 1998). Whilst most psychological interventions are aimed at improving well-being by reducing emotional dysregulation, CBT approaches seek to help people manage incoming perceptual stimuli and mediate the frequency, intensity, duration and level of emotional arousal a person experiences (Papa, Boland and Sewell 2012). Historically, CBT has employed strategies to help people identify and accept their current emotions and to change current emotional reactions (Fruzzetti et al. 2008). Examples of these could include helping people to discriminate between their emotions and accurate labelling of emotional experience, and developing strategies for changing emotional reactions, by stepping back from inner experiences and managing automatic thoughts. Building on these ideas, contemporary CBT approaches often seek to help people to develop strategies to self-regulate attentional focus on present moment experiencing. This present moment focus, coupled with acceptance of emotional response, is intended to help people connect with current emotions and experiences, increase tolerance to those emotions and reduce emotional avoidance (Papa, Boland and Sewell 2012). Examples of emotional regulation focused interventions can include mindfulness techniques (Segal, Williams and Teasdale 2013), strategies to tackle experiential avoidance (Harris 2006) and grounding techniques (Fisher 1999). The evidence for the effectiveness of CBT in promoting emotional regulation and the benefits of improving emotional regulation is accumulating. A recent meta-analysis concluded that CBT approaches can help people to reduce avoidance of difficult emotions and troubling thoughts, whilst promoting active engagement with emotional experiencing and reducing tendencies to reinforce heightened negative emotions (Daros et al. 2021). CBT approaches therefore can help people to balance emotional and cognitive processing of experience.

Future Directions in CBT Research and Practice

CBT approaches have established themselves not only as effective treatments for mental health distress, but also for promoting quality of life and psychological well-being for people experiencing difficult circumstances or physical illness (Beck 2019). The success of CBT approaches derives from their strong grounding in psychological theory, their heavy emphasis on therapist and client creating a warm, empathic and respectful therapeutic relationship and their commitment to scientific evaluation of therapy efficacy and effectiveness (Kennerely et al. 2020). These strengths have supported CBT approaches in moving beyond treating distress, towards promoting positive mental health and well-being. Increasingly, applications of CBT approaches to promote well-being can be seen in the literature. Examples include adapting CBT approaches to support adolescents who have experienced bullying (Lydecker 2022), managing school-based stress (Ulaş and Seçer 2022) and preventing depression (Hetrick et al. 2016). Alongside these applications of CBT approaches, contemporary developments in CBT research are progressively focusing towards adaptive functioning in the presence of adversity and pursuing meaningful and enjoyable life, despite significant personal, interpersonal or contextual challenges (Beck, Finkel and Beck 2021). CBT approaches to health promotion are not about ignoring socio-economic or other problems but validating experience and fostering a sense of control with appropriate reactions in context, to promote a healthier sense of self. CBT approaches, therefore, have a role to play alongside other public health approaches to mental health promotion.

Conclusion

In this chapter, we have seen the increasing need for MHP, with the numbers of young people seeking support increasing. As we emerge from the Covid-19 pandemic, there appears to be unprecedented stress and strain on mental health services, and at a time when structural determinants of mental health are becoming increasingly visible, such as the impact of widening inequality. MHP interventions can occur across structural, societal and individual levels. Psychological interventions, in particular CBT approaches, are important at the individual level for promoting well-being. CBT approaches can work alongside wider structural and societal interventions as part of a layered approach to MHP.

References

Alegría, M., NeMoyer, A., Falgàs Bagué, I., Wang, Y. and Alvarez, K. (2018). Social determinants of mental health: Where we are and where we need to go. *Current Psychiatry Reports*, 20(11), p. 95. 10.1007/s11920-018-0969-9.

American Psychological Association. (2022). *Resilience*. Washington DC: American Psychological Association. Available at: https://dictionary.apa.org/resilience [accessed 30.09.2022]

Appleby, J. (2019). Nursing workforce crisis in numbers. *British Medical Journal (Online)*, 367. https://doi.org/10.1136/bmj.l6664.

Bailey, A.M. (2020). Psychiatric formulation and the structural determinants of mental health. *Academic Psychiatry*, 44(6), pp. 804–805. 10.1007/s40596-020-01307-9.

Bannister, R. (2021). Underfunded mental healthcare in the NHS: The cycle of preventable distress continues. *BMJ*, 375, n2706. https://doi.org/10.1136/bmj.n2706

Baxter, A.J., Scott, K.M., Ferrari, A.J., Norman, R.E., Vos, T. and Whiteford, H.A. (2014). Challenging the myth of an "epidemic" of common mental disorders: Trends in the global prevalence of anxiety and depression between 1990 and 2010. *Depression and Anxiety*, 31(6), pp. 506–516. https://doi.org/10.1002/da.22230.

Beck, A.T. (1963). Thinking and depression: I. Idiosyncratic content and cognitive distortions. *Archives of General Psychiatry*, 9(4), pp. 324–333. 10.1001/archpsyc.1963.01720160014002.

Beck, A.T. (1976). *Cognitive therapy and the emotional disorders*. London: Penguin.

Beck, A.T. (1997). The past and future of cognitive therapy. *Journal of Psychotherapy Practice and Research*, 6(4), pp. 276–84.

Beck, A.T. (2019). A 60-year evolution of cognitive theory and therapy. *Perspectives on Psychological Science*, 14(1), pp. 16–20. 10.1177/1745691618804187.

Beck, A.T., Finkel, M.R. and Beck, J.S. (2021) The theory of modes: Applications to schizophrenia and other psychological conditions. *Cognitive Therapy and Research*, 45(3), pp. 391–400. 10.1007/s10608-020-10098-0.

Bennett, M.P., Knight, R., Patel, S., So, T., Dunning, D., Barnhofer, T., Smith, P., Kuyken, W., Ford, T. and Dalgleish, T. (2021). Decentering as a core component in the psychological treatment and prevention of youth anxiety and depression: A narrative review and insight report. *Translational Psychiatry*, 11(1), p. 288. 10.1038/s41398-021-01397-5.

Bernstein, A., Hadash, Y., Lichtash, Y., Tanay, G., Shepherd, K. and Fresco, D.M. (2015). Decentering and related constructs: A critical review and metacognitive processes model. *Perspectives on Psychological Science*, 10(5), pp. 599–617. 10.1177/1745691615594577.

Centre for Disease Control and Prevention. (2022). *What is children's mental health?* Atlanta, GA: U.S. Department of Health & Human Services. Available at: https://www.cdc.gov/childrensmental health/basics.html#print [accessed 04.10.2022].

Compton, M.T. and Shim, R.S. (2015). The social determinants of mental health. *Focus*, 13, pp. 419–425. doi: 10.1176/appi.focus.20150017.

Cybulski, L., Ashcroft, D.M., Carr, M.J., Garg, S., Chew-Graham, C.A., Kapur, N. and Webb, R.T. (2021). Temporal trends in annual incidence rates for psychiatric disorders and self-harm among children and adolescents in the UK, 2003–2018. *BMC Psychiatry*, 21(1), p. 229. 10.1186/s12888-021-03235-w.

Daros, A.R., Haefner, S.A., Asadi, S., Kazi, S., Rodak, T. and Quilty, L.C. (2021). A meta-analysis of emotional regulation outcomes in psychological interventions for youth with depression and anxiety. *Nature Human Behaviour*, 5(10), pp. 1443–1457. 10.1038/s41562-021-01191-9.

David, D., Cristea, I. and Hofmann, S.G. (2018). Why cognitive behavioral therapy is the current gold standard of psychotherapy. *Frontiers in Psychiatry*, 9(4). 10.3389/fpsyt.2018.00004.

Denckla, C.A., Cicchetti, D., Kubzansky, L.D., Seedat, S., Teicher, M.H., Williams, D.R. and Koenen, K.C. (2020). Psychological resilience: An update on definitions, a critical appraisal, and research recommendations. *European Journal of Psychotraumatology*, 11(1), 1822064. 10.1080/20008198. 2020.1822064.

Dragioti, E., Li, H., Tsitsas, G., Lee, K.H., Choi, J., Kim, J., Choi, Y.J., Tsamakis, K., Estradé, A., Agorastos, A., Vancampfort, D., Tsiptsios, D., Thompson, T., Mosina, A., Vakadaris, G., Fusar-Poli, P., Carvalho, A.F., Correll, C.U., Han, Y.J., Park, S., Il Shin, J. and Solmi, M. (2022). A large-scale meta-analytic atlas of mental health problems prevalence during the COVID-19 early pandemic. *Journal of Medical Virology*, 94(5), pp. 1935–1949. https://doi.org/10.1002/jmv.27549.

Engel, G. (1977). The need for a new medical model: A challenge for biomedicine. *Science*, 196, pp. 129–136. https://science.sciencemag.org/content/196/4286/129.

Faculty of Public Health and Mental Health Foundation. (2016). *Better mental health for all: A public health approach to mental health improvement*. London: Faculty of Public Health.

Fisher, J. (1999). *The work of stabilization in trauma treatment*. Unpublished paper presented at The Trauma Center Lecture Series, Boston, MA.

Fruzzetti, A.E., Crook, W., Erikson, K.M., Lee, J.E. and Worrall, J.M. (2008). Emotion regulation. In: O'Donohue, W. and Fisher, J.E., eds. *Cognitive behavior therapy: Applying empirically supported techniques in your practice*. Hoboken, NJ: John Wiley.

Gloster, A.T., Meyer, A.H. and Lieb, R. (2017). Psychological flexibility as a malleable public health target: Evidence from a representative sample. *Journal of Contextual Behavioral Science*, 6(2), pp. 166–171. https://doi.org/10.1016/j.jcbs.2017.02.003.

Gross, J.J. (1998). The emerging field of emotion regulation: An integrative review. *Review of General Psychology*, 2(3), pp. 271–299. 10.1037/1089-2680.2.3.271.

Harris, R. (2006). Embracing your demons: An overview of acceptance and commitment therapy. *Psychotherapy in Australia*, 12(4), pp. 2–8.

Hetrick, S.E., Cox, G.R., Witt, K.G., Bir, J.J. and Merry, S.N. (2016). Cognitive behavioural therapy (CBT), third-wave CBT and interpersonal therapy (IPT) based interventions for preventing depression in children and adolescents. *Cochrane Database of Systematic Reviews* (8). 10.1002/14651858. CD003380.pub4.

Hofmann, S.G., Asmundson, G.J.G. and Beck, A.T. (2013). The science of cognitive therapy. *Behavior Therapy*, 44(2), pp. 199–212. https://doi.org/10.1016/j.beth.2009.01.007.

Huppert, F.A. (2009). Psychological well-being: Evidence regarding its causes and consequences. *Applied Psychology: Health and Well-Being*, 1(2), pp. 137–164. https://doi.org/10.1111/j.1758-0854.2009.01008.x.

Institute of Medicine Committee on Prevention of Mental Disorders. (1994). In: Mrazek, P.J. & Haggerty, R.J., eds. *Reducing risks for mental disorders: Frontiers for preventive intervention research*. Washington (DC): National Academies Press (US).

Jané-Llopis, E., Barry, M., Hosman, C. and Patel, V. (2005). Mental health promotion works: A review. *Promotion & Education*, 12(suppl 2), pp. 9–25. 10.1177/10253823050120020103x.

Kashdan, T.B. and Rottenberg, J. (2010). Psychological flexibility as a fundamental aspect of health. *Clinical Psychology Review*, 30(7), pp. 865–878. https://doi.org/10.1016/j.cpr.2010.03.001.

Kennerely, H., Butler, G., Fennell, M. and Rakovshik, S. (2020). Twenty-five years of CBT: An OCTC perspective. *CBT Today*, 48(1), pp. 20–22.

Kobau, R., Seligman, M.E., Peterson, C., Diener, E., Zack, M.M., Chapman, D. and Thompson, W. (2011). Mental health promotion in public health: Perspectives and strategies from positive psychology. *American Journal of Public Health*, 101(8), p. e1–9. 10.2105/ajph.2010.300083.

Liberati, E., Richards, N., Willars, J., Scott, D., Boydell, N., Parker, J., Pinfold, V., Martin, G., Dixon-Woods, M. and Jones, P.B. (2021). A qualitative study of experiences of NHS mental healthcare workers during the covid-19 pandemic. *BMC Psychiatry*, 21(1), p. 250. 10.1186/s12888-021-03261-8.

Lucas, J.J. and Moore, K.A. (2019). Psychological flexibility: Positive implications for mental health and life satisfaction. *Health Promotion International*, 35(2), pp. 312–320. 10.1093/heapro/daz036.

Lydecker, J.A. (2022). Conceptual application of trauma-focused cognitive behavioral therapy to treat victims of bullying. *Journal of Prevention and Health Promotion*, 3(2), pp. 231–245. 10.1177/26320770221074008.

Marmot, M., Allen, J., Boyce, T., Goldblatt, P. and Morrison, J. (2020). *Health equity in England: The marmot review 10 years on*. London: Institute of Health Equity.

Marmot, M., Allen, J., Goldblatt, P., Boyce, T., McNeish, D., Grady, M. and Geddes, I. (2010). *Fair society, healthy lives: The Marmot Review*. London: Strategic Review of Health Inequalities in England post-2010.

McMain, S., Newman, M.G., Segal, Z.V. and DeRubeis, R.J. (2015). Cognitive behavioral therapy: Current status and future research directions. *Psychotherapy Research*, 25(3), pp. 321–329. 10.1080/10503307.2014.1002440.

Newman, K.L., Jeve, Y. and Majumder, P. (2022). Experiences and emotional strain of NHS frontline workers during the peak of the COVID-19 pandemic. *International Journal of Social Psychiatry*, 68(4), pp. 783–790. 10.1177/00207640211006153.

NHS providers. (2017). *The state of the NHS provider sector*. London: NHS providers.

O'Connor, M., Arnup, S.J., Mensah, F., Olsson, C., Goldfeld, S., Viner, R.M. and Hope, S. (2022). Natural history of mental health competence from childhood to adolescence. *Journal of Epidemiology and Community Health*, 76(2), pp. 133–139. 10.1136/jech-2021-216761.

Palmer, B. and Rolewicz, L. (2022). *Peak leaving? A spotlight on nurse leaver rates in the UK*. London: The Nuffield Trust. Available at: https://www.nuffieldtrust.org.uk/resource/peak-leaving-a-spotlight-on-nurse-leaver-rates-in-the-uk

Papa, A., Boland, M. and Sewell, M.T. (2012). Emotion regulation and CBT. In: O'Donohue, W. and Fisher, J.E., eds. *Cognitive behavior therapy*. Hoboken, NJ: Wiley.

Patel, K., Robertson, E., Kwong, A.S.F., Griffith, G.J., Willan, K., Green, M.J., Di Gessa, G., Huggins, C.F., McElroy, E., Thompson, E.J., Maddock, J., Niedzwiedz, C.L., Henderson, M., Richards, M., Steptoe, A., Ploubidis, G.B., Moltrecht, B., Booth, C., Fitzsimons, E., Silverwood, R., Patalay, P., Porteous, D. and Katikireddi, S.V. (2022). Psychological distress before and during the COVID-19 pandemic among adults in the United Kingdom based on coordinated analyses of 11 longitudinal studies. *JAMA Network Open*, 5(4), pp. e227629–e227629. 10.1001/jamanetworkopen.2022.7629.

Plewes, J. (2022). *Analysis: The rise in mental health demand*. London: NHS confederation. Available at: https://www.nhsconfed.org/articles/analysis-rise-mental-health-demand#:~:text=Rising%20demand&text=In%20terms%20of%20activity%2C%20in,to%20the%20pandemic%20(2%2C131%2C113)

Purgato, M., Uphoff, E., Singh, R., Thapa Pachya, A., Abdulmalik, J. and van Ginneken, N. (2020). Promotion, prevention and treatment interventions for mental health in low- and middle-income countries through a task-shifting approach. *Epidemiology and Psychiatric Sciences*, 29, p. e150. 10.1017/S204579602000061X.

Racine, N., McArthur, B.A., Cooke, J.E., Eirich, R., Zhu, J. and Madigan, S. (2021). Global prevalence of depressive and anxiety symptoms in children and adolescents during COVID-19: A meta-analysis. *JAMA Pediatrics*, 175(11), pp. 1142–1150. 10.1001/jamapediatrics.2021.2482.

Royal College of Paediatrics and Child Health. (2020). *State of child health*. London: Royal College of Paediatrics and Child Health.

Salkovskis, P.M. (2002). Empirically grounded clinical interventions: Cognitive-behavioural therapy progresses through a multi-dimensional approach to clinical science. *Behavioural and Cognitive Psychotherapy*, 30(1), pp. 3–9. 10.1017/S1352465802001029.

Segal, Z.V., Williams, J.M.G. and Teasdale, J.D. (2013). *Mindfulness-based cognitive therapy for depression*. 2nd ed. New York, NY: The Guilford Press.

Shevlin, M., Butter, S., McBride, O., Murphy, J., Gibson-Miller, J., Hartman, T.K., Levita, L., Mason, L., Martinez, A.P., McKay, R., Stocks, T.V.A., Bennett, K., Hyland, P. and Bentall, R.P. (2021). Refuting the myth of a 'tsunami' of mental ill-health in populations affected by COVID-19: Evidence that response to the pandemic is heterogeneous, not homogeneous. *Psychological Medicine*, 1–9. 10.1017/S0033291721001665.

Slee, A., Nazareth, I., Freemantle, N. and Horsfall, L. (2021). Trends in generalised anxiety disorders and symptoms in primary care: UK population-based cohort study. *The British Journal of Psychiatry*, 218(3), pp. 158–164. 10.1192/bjp.2020.159.

Stott, R., Mansell, W., Salkovskis, P., Lavender, A. and Cartwright-Hatton, S. (2010). *Oxford guide to metaphors in CBT*. Oxford: Oxford University Press.

Thapar, A., Eyre, O., Patel, V. and Brent, D. (2022). Depression in young people. *The Lancet*, 400(10352), pp. 617–631. https://doi.org/10.1016/S0140-6736(22)01012-1.

Twenge, J.M., Cooper, A.B., Joiner, T.E., Duffy, M.E. and Binau, S.G. (2019). Age, period, and cohort trends in mood disorder indicators and suicide-related outcomes in a nationally representative dataset, 2005–2017. *Journal of Abnormal Psychology*, 128, pp. 185–199. 10.1037/abn0000410.

Ulaş, S. and Seçer, İ. (2022). Developing a CBT-based intervention program for reducing school burnout and investigating its effectiveness with mixed methods research. *Frontiers in Psychology*, 13. 10.3389/fpsyg.2022.884912.

United Nations. (2013). *Definition of youth*. New York: United Nations. Available at: https://www.un.org/esa/socdev/documents/youth/fact-sheets/youth-definition.pdf

United Nations. (2020). *Policy brief: COVID-19 and the need for action on mental health*. Geneva: United Nations. Available at: https://unsdg.un.org/resources/policy-brief-covid-19-and-need-action-mental-health

United Nations. (2022a). *Children*. New York, NY: United Nations. Available at: https://www.un.org/en/global-issues/children

United Nations. (2022b). *Youth*. New York, NY: United Nations. Available at: https://www.un.org/en/global-issues/youth

United Nations Children's Fund. (2021). *The state of the world's children 2021: On my mind – Promoting, protecting and caring for children's mental health*. New York, NY: UNICEF.

Wilkinson, E. (2015). UK NHS staff: Stressed, exhausted, burnt out. *The Lancet*, 385(9971), pp. 841–842. https://doi.org/10.1016/S0140-6736(15)60470-6.

Wilkinson, R. and Pickett, K. (2009). *The spirit level: Why more equal societies almost always do better*. London: Penguin.

Wills, F. and Sanders, D. (2013). *Cognitive behaviour therapy: Foundations for practice*. 3rd ed. London: Sage.

World Health Organization. (2004). Prevention of Mental Disorders: Effective Interventions and Policy Options: Summary report/A report of the World Health Organization, Department of Mental Health and Substance Abuse in collaboration with the Prevention Research Centre of the Universities of Nijmegen and Maastricht. Geneva. Available at: https://apps.who.int/iris/handle/10665/43027

World Health Organization. (2021). *Adolescent mental health*. Available at: https://www.who.int/news-room/fact-sheets/detail/adolescent-mental-health

World Health Organization. (2022). *Mental health: Strengthening our response*. Geneva: World Health Organization. Available at: https://www.who.int/news-room/fact-sheets/detail/mental-health-strengthening-our-response

World Health Organization and Calouste Gulbenkian Foundation. (2014). *Social determinants of mental health*. Geneva: World Health Organization.

11 Promoting the Health of People with a Learning Disability

David Charnock

Introduction

This chapter will assist anyone working to promote health and to work more effectively with people who have a learning disability. Its aim is to offer a clear definition of this complex spectrum of disabilities to improve understanding and to provide the foundation on which to build a strategy to promote positive health outcomes for this group of people.

Currently, there are no precise statistics on the number of people with a learning disability living in the UK. According to Mencap (undated), 2.16% (approximately 1.1 million) adults have a learning disability in the UK and 2.5% of children also have a learning disability. Although it is apparent that this group makes up only a small percentage of the population, they are known to have significantly disproportionate problems with their health compared to the general population. As such, they often require significant and long-term support to maintain good health and benefit from the same health outcomes as the general population (Public Health England 2018).

It is critical that those working in health promotion or who have this as an aspect of their work consider the needs of people with a learning disability carefully to ensure that they have equitable access to health promotion and health care. According to NHS Digital (2020), the current life expectancy for men with a learning disability is 14 years below the general population and for a woman with a learning disability, it is 17 years. In 2021, almost 50% of the deaths of people who had a learning disability were considered 'avoidable', compared to just over 20% of the general population (White et al. 2022). The causes of 'avoidable' death for people who have a learning disability are mostly related to cancer, hypertension, diabetes and respiratory conditions. Many of these 'avoidable' deaths are due, in part, to a lack of reasonable adjustment in health services. It is critical that those working to promote the health of this population understand that these adjustments can make the difference between the person continuing to live a full and meaningful life or having that life cut short.

The following section will help you to clearly define learning disability and learn how adjustments can be made to help promote good health. It will also help you to consider how best to create a strategy for health promotion with people who have a learning disability, their allies and caregivers.

Defining Issues of Health and Health Promotion for Learning Disability Practice

Definition

Learning disability is often used homogeneously to describe what is in fact a complex group of heterogeneous conditions caused by a number of prenatal, perinatal and postnatal factors.

DOI: 10.4324/9781003411321-11

These include chromosome and genetic anomalies, maternal infection, early or prolonged labour, prematurity or environmental/social factors. It is widely thought that the principal criterion for recognising someone with a learning disability is a lower intellectual ability, but it is necessary to establish this only after a detailed understanding of the person is made. In UK health services, a learning disability is contextualised as including three interconnected factors: 'a significantly reduced ability to understand new or complex information; to learn new skills (impaired intelligence); a reduced ability to cope independently (impaired social functioning)' (National Institute for Health and Care Excellence 2022). To be regarded as a person with a learning disability, all three factors have to be present before adulthood and have a lasting effect on development. It is essential to recognise that despite the identification of these factors, a person with a learning disability is able to cope with new information, learn skills and be independent. However, additional supports and adjustments will often be required to help the individual exercise their rights, take control of their lives and be included as part of their community.

Health and Co-morbidities

In addition to 'avoidable deaths' in people with a learning disability in the UK, there are a number of co-morbidities affecting the lives of this group (see Perera et al. 2019). Those working to promote health should be aware of these and the social determinants that also significantly affect people with a learning disability. Figure 11.1 shows the common co-morbidities and social determinants that impact the lives of this group.

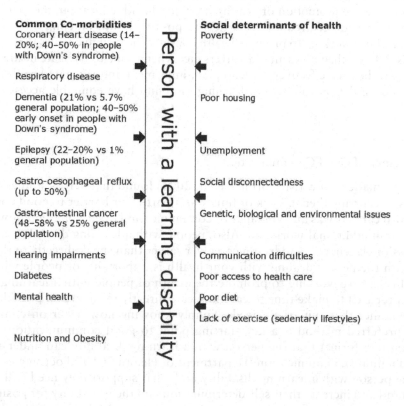

Figure 11.1 Common Co-morbidities and the Social Determinants of Health for People Who Have a Learning Disability

It is critical that those who work to promote the health of people with a learning disability are cognisant of the common health issues and the socio-structural factors that impact the health of this group. These issues and factors should influence the strategy for health promotion plans and activities to positively affect health outcomes.

Health checks and good support networks can mitigate the effects of poor health and the socio-structural impacts of living as part of society. This has long been recommended, although the research on their effective uptake is small (Macdonald et al. 2018; McConkey, Taggart and Kane 2015; Michell 2012). These health checks could offer an opportunity for those with responsibility for health promotion to evaluate and establish clear outcomes for their interventions.

Equitable Access to Health Care

It is important to recognise that people with learning disabilities require adjustments to navigate both the physical health environment and the cognitive aspects of building and maintaining good health. Roll (2018), in their conceptual analysis, recognised that two aspects act as antecedents to the health promotion of people who have a learning disability. These are access to health care and the health providers focus on the disability and not the person. It is possible that these antecedents can combine to form systemic barriers that cause problems for people with a learning disability, their allies and caregivers. Roll (2018) goes on to locate the promotion of healthy lifestyles, health education, the involvement of supporters and person centredness as critical to positive health outcomes. It is, therefore, essential that those working to promote health consider the systemic issues that people with learning disabilities, their allies and caregivers face when trying to navigate health care. This knowledge can be used effectively to help plan, implement and evaluate health-promotion activity, ensuring that people with a learning disability have equitable access to support good health.

The Importance of Good Communication

A recent systematic review (McCormick et al. 2021) found that across studies communication was a recurring theme. Lack of time was a particular barrier to good communication in health care, as was an avoidance of communication due to limited knowledge and concerns about additional workload. Also, people with a learning disability were aware that professionals tended to address a caregiver rather than speak directly to them. Being familiar with the person dealing with your health is important for people with a learning disability. Those working to promote the health of people with a learning disability should be prepared to make time to communicate directly to them and provide information in a manner that suits their needs. Simply knowing how a person communicates and their preferred method is a key starting point to good communication. Providing information in a format that the person with a learning disability can understand is essential to facilitate communication (Department of Health 2010). Focusing communication on the person with a learning disability and what support they need will help them to understand and increase their self-determination and the possibility for positive health outcomes.

Critical Thinking

Take time to research and consider the following.

As you begin to learn more about the complexities of health for people with a learning disability, pause and think about the following critical questions:

What can those working to promote health do to include people with learning disabilities in decisions about health promotion activity?

How might those working to promote health balance the need to direct health promotion activity for people with learning disabilities with the need for self-determination and choice?

Building a Strategy for Health Promotion with People Who Have a Learning Disability

In this section, the work of Beattie (1991) is used to suggest a foundation from which a strategy for health promotion can be built for people with a learning disability. My focus here is to ensure that in all aspects of the creation of strategy, the person with a learning disability is central, allowing for good decisions that promote autonomy. Approaches to the support of people with a learning disability have a long history of control and paternalism. The advent of normalisation policies across the world has helped to increase opportunities for person centred approaches to care and opportunities for self-determination. These approaches in more contemporary times jar with reports of the untimely deaths of people who have a learning disability from preventable illness and unequal access to health care systems in the UK. Beattie's (1991) work offers a framework to help scrutinise the role of the state and community in the promotion of health for people with a learning disability and form a foundation on which to build a strategy. In addition, it offers an opportunity to consider the changing roles of professionals, allies and caregivers in the lives of this group. In this section, I would like to use Beattie's (1991) work to establish a set of points of reflection for those working in health promotion, to be able to scrutinise 'Expertise', 'Policy', 'User voice' and 'Collective action'. Figure 11.2 is an attempt to summarise the reference points for questions about the development of a strategy for health promotion. Unlike Beattie's (1991) structural map, which attempted to extract the clashes between structures of accountability in health promotion strategy, this adaptation aims to help health promotion professionals make sense of the lives of people with a learning disability to promote health. It is the synergy between the person with a learning disability, their allies and caregivers, the professional in health promotion and the policy landscape that will help to determine a clear strategy for health promotion work.

The following presents an account of how each quadrant in Figure 11.2 should be approached. At the end of each of the sections, I present suggestions for key strategic questions that could be used to formulate the foundation for a health promotion strategy for working with an individual or group with learning disabilities.

Health Persuasions 'Expertise'

Although Beattie (1991) regarded this as raising questions of paternalism in health promotion, an alternative view is proposed for those working with people who have a learning

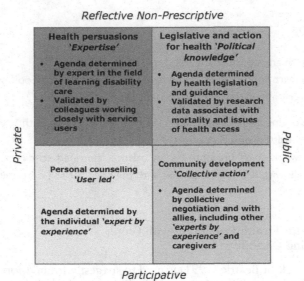

Figure 11.2 Strategy Building Adapted from Beattie (1991)

disability. In this quadrant, strategic questions should be raised about the intervention of the professional and how their expertise should be used in relation to health promotion and the individual or group. It is important to recognise the role of those working closely with the individual or group to determine a more complete picture of their health needs. This should be done in a reflective and non-prescriptive way to establish how we know something and if this knowledge is still accurate. Those working in health promotion should work alongside 'experts' in learning disability practice to develop their knowledge of the health needs of the person or group of people with learning disabilities. They should then validate this new knowledge by talking to people who know the person or group well to correct any assumption made.

Key strategic questions

- What is already known about the health of people who have a learning disability?
- What evidence will help to support change for the individual or group?
- Who are the key collaborators?

Legislative and Action for Health 'Policy'

In Beattie's (1991) work, this quadrant was regarded as imposing bureaucratic control and scientific authority on strategy for health, far removed from the person. In this adaptation, it is the importance of the health issue and how access to health care services and considerations of mortality are utilised to shape strategic questions about the promotion of health for the individual. As mentioned previously, there are significant issues with both life expectancy and mortality that in some cases should influence decisions about health and health promotion. Therefore, any risk of bureaucratic interference is neutralised by the need to incorporate knowledge of specific threats to health and well-being emerging from policy or action for health. Without this wider political view, it is difficult to know how to positively impact the health of people with learning disabilities.

Key strategic questions

- Which current national legislation or guidance can help us formulate a plan for change?
- Do national/local guides or programmes exist that can be adapted to help facilitate the development of a programme of health promotion?

Personal Counselling 'User Voice'

Beattie (1991) regarded this as the domain of the person with regard to decisions about their health and self-determination. For all people who have a learning disability, this should be an essential part of strategic questioning prior to planning health promotion activity. Assumptions should not be made about an individual's ability to make decisions about their health without a complete discussion with them and the people who know them best. This will again help to establish what supports are necessary and how to introduce reasonable adjustments to communication and information to allow the person to participate as fully as possible.

Key strategic questions

- How does the person or group experience health?
- What barriers to health promotion currently exist for the service user?

Community Development 'Collective Action'

Here Beattie (1991) focussed on the collective work of allies to determine the strategy for health promotion. People who have a learning disability can have many allies or only a few, but these allies can play a significant part in the health of the individual and the successful outcome of health-related work. It would, therefore, be essential to establish a clear working relationship with allies to assist in the development of a clear strategy for health promotion. As a consequence of relationship building in this way, it may be possible for health promotion professionals to see more clearly the possibility for collective action on specific health issues for people who have a learning disability, with particular reference to those which have resulted in premature death for this population. This quadrant is particularly significant as it includes the voices of other *'Experts by experience'* to ground health promotion strategy in the lives of this community.

Key strategic questions

- Who do the individual or group regard as their allies?
- What do allies and caregivers say about health?
- How are allies and caregivers currently supporting the health of the individual or group?

Activity: Applying Beattie's (1991) work to shape strategy for health promotion for people who have a learning disability

There are numerous aspects of health that could be considered by health promotion practitioners for action. Many of these can initially be decided upon by further analysing the co-morbidities and social determinants that impact the lives of this group. It is essential that practitioners begin with a clear strategy to help secure positive outcomes for people who have a learning disability.

To help demonstrate this, one aspect of health has been chosen with the potential to effect positive outcome on morbidity and co-morbidities for this group. Diaz (2020) identifies physical activity as the main priority for health promotion practitioners working with people who have a learning disability. In their analysis of seven waves of a national survey in the United Stated, Diaz (2020) was able to identify a positive effect on mortality and co-morbidities for people with a learning disability. In an earlier Australian study, Koritsas and Iacono (2016) also identify physical activity and healthy eating as priorities for health promotion activity for people with a learning disability. The following uses Beattie's (1991) work, adapted for this group in Figure 11.1, to begin to build a strategy on which to base an approach to health promotion to begin to increase physical activity for people who have a learning disability. The reader is asked to address the critical question at the end of each section to further build the strategy. The answers can be extracted from the information in the sections above.

Health Persuasions 'Expertise'

Beginning with specific issues with mortality, the co-morbidities which are associated with this group and the determinants that have a particular impact on their lives, we can begin to establish a clear foundation for any plans to promote good health. Harnessing evidence about inactivity amongst the general population can be further enhanced by using research evidence on this population to offer a clear direction for the strategy we are beginning to build. For example, Melville et al. (2018), in the first population-based study of its kind, found that higher levels of sedentary behaviour were evident in the lives of people with a learning disability when compared to the general population. On this basis, the researchers support behaviour changing programmes for people with a learning disability to prevent sedentary lifestyle. Evidence like this can help to build a picture of the specific health issues and how best to address them using the available expertise.

Critical Question

What knowledge would you need about the communication needs of people with a learning disability?

Legislative and Action for Health 'Political Knowledge'

Knowledge of legislation or guidance about health is essential to ensure that people who have a learning disability are included. Remembering to incorporate guidance for all citizens about health as well as that specifically written or adapted for people with a learning disability is important to ensure that they have equitable access to support. Increasing physical activity for people with a learning disability allows for consideration of mainstream guidance released by the Chief Medical Officer for the UK (Department of Health and Social Care, Llwodraeth Cymru Welsh Government, Department of Health Northern Ireland

and the Scottish Government 2019), adapting this to meet the needs of people with learning disabilities. In addition, using guides from charitable organisations (Mencap 2020) can be a useful addition, providing accessible guidance for the person, their allies and caregivers. The important thing here is that national guidance, including those rooted in legislation, can help to strengthen a strategy to address issues specific to the health of people with a learning disability.

Critical Question

Why is mortality such a significant issue for people with a learning disability and how can a health promotion strategy help?

Personal Counselling 'User Led'

Having contact with the person or group of people with a learning disability will ensure that the strategy is person centred. Understanding health needs will also help to shape the strategy to accommodate idiosyncrasies and personal preference in relation to physical activity. Starting with the person themselves will help to challenge the barriers that often lie in the way of behavioural change in relation to sedentary lifestyles. One barrier identified by Cartwright, Reid and Hammersley (2016) was the restriction put on activities by carers as a result of their own preference and limited resources. Starting to build strategy with the person or group of people with a learning disability will help to identify limitations and their own personal preferences first. As discussed earlier in this chapter, finding the best way to communicate with people with a learning disability will be critical to ensuring that their voice is heard through the strategy.

Critical Question

What specific barriers or antecedents might people with a learning disability face and how can these be addressed?

Community Development 'Collective Action'

The characteristics of support professionals and family caregivers can have an impact on increasing physical activity for people who have a learning disability (Bossink et al. 2019; Cartwright, Reid and Hammersley 2016). It is, therefore, critical when developing a strategy for health promotion activity with people with a learning disability that you involve those individuals who support them in their lives. This should not be exclusively limited to family members or paid caregivers; there may also be friends and other users by experience who have ideas to offer. The critical point here is that the health promotion professional should join with others in collective action to improve health outcomes for the individual or group. Without this collaborative approach, it is likely that health promotion activity will not be successful.

Critical Question

Why are caregivers important to the building of successful strategy for health promotion?

Key Messages

The key principles for working with people with learning disabilities to build strategies for health promotion are as follows:

- **Be clear** about the health needs of people with learning disabilities in relation to mortality and co-morbidities.
- **Understand and adjust** to the communication needs of people with learning disabilities and make room for independence and self-determination.
- **Don't assume** what people with a learning disability will understand, get to know them first.
- **Collaborate** with others to create a clear strategy for health promotion that is suited to the needs of people with a learning disability.

References

Beattie, A. (1991). Knowledge and control in health promotion: A test case for social policy and social theory. In: Gabe, J., Calnan, M. and Bury, M., eds. *The sociology of the health service*. London: Routledge, pp. 162–202.

Bossink, L.W.M., van der Outten, A.A.J., Paap, M.C.S. and Vlaskamp, C. (2019). Factors associated with direct support professionals' behaviour in the physical activity support provided to people with intellectual disabilities. *Journal of Intellectual Disability Research*, 63(8), pp. 981–999.

Cartwright, L., Reid, M. and Hammersley, R. (2016). Barriers to increasing the physical activity of people with intellectual disabilities. *British Journal of Learning Disabilities*, 45, pp. 47–55.

Department of Health. (2010). *Making written information easier to understand for people with learning disabilities* [online]. Available at: https://assets.publishing.service.gov.uk/government/uploads/system/uploads/attachment_data/file/215923/dh_121927.pdf

Department of Health and Social Care, Llwodraeth Cymru Welsh Government, Department of Health Northern Ireland and the Scottish Government. (2019). *UK Chief Medical Officers' physical activity guidelines* [online]. Available at: https://assets.publishing.service.gov.uk/government/uploads/system/uploads/attachment_data/file/832868/uk-chief-medical-officers-physical-activity-guidelines.pdf

Diaz, K.M. (2020). Leisure-time physical activity and all-cause mortality among adults with intellectual disability: The national health interview survey. *Journal of Intellectual Disability Research*, 64(2), pp. 180–184.

Koritsas, S. and Iacono, T. (2016). Weight, nutrition, food choice, and physical activity in adults with intellectual disability. *Journal of Intellectual Disability Research*, 60(4), pp. 355–364.

Macdonald, S., Morrison, J., Melville, C.A., Baltzer, M., MacArthur, L. and Cooper, S.A. (2018). Embedding routine health checks for adults with intellectual disabilities in primary care: Practice nurse perceptions. *Journal of Intellectual Disability Research*, 62(4), pp. 349–357.

McConkey, R., Taggart, L. and Kane, M. (2015). Optimizing the uptake of health checks for people with intellectual disabilities. *Journal of Intellectual Disabilities*, 19(3), pp. 205–214.

McCormick, F., March, L., Taggart, L. and Brown, M. (2021). Experiences of adults with intellectual disabilities accessing acute hospital services: A systematic review of the international evidence. Health and Social Care in the Community, 29, pp. 1222–1232.

Melville, C.A., McGarty, A., Harris, L., Baltzer, M., McArthur, L.A., Morrison, J., Allan, L. and Cooper, S.A. (2018). A population-based, cross sectional study of the prevalence and correlated of sedentary behaviour of adults with intellectual disabilities. *Journal of Intellectual Disability Research*, 62(1), pp. 60–71.

Mencap. (undated). *Research statistics* [online]. Available at: https://www.mencap.org.uk/learning-disability-explained/research-and-statistics#:~:text=There%20are%201.5%20million%20people,to%20finding%20work%20and%20friendships.

Mencap. (2020). *Lets' Get Active: A guide to physical activity and sport for people with a learning disability*. Available at: https://www.mencap.org.uk/sites/default/files/2020-07/2020.162%20 Lets%20Get%20Active%20-%20Easy%20Read.pdf

Michell, B. (2012). Checking up on Des: My life my choice's research into annual health checks for people with learning disabilities in Oxfordshire. *British Journal of Learning Disabilities*, 40, pp. 152–161.

National Institute for Health and Care Excellence. (2022). *Learning disabilities: What is it?* Available at: https://cks.nice.org.uk/topics/learning-disabilities/background-information/definition/

NHS Digital. (2020). *Health and care of people with learning disabilities, experimental statistics: 2018 to 2019* [online]. Available at: https://digital.nhs.uk/data-and-information/publications/ statistical/health-and-care-of-people-with-learning-disabilities/experimental-statistics-2018-to-2019/condition-prevalence

Perera, B., Audi, S., Solomou, S., Courteney, K. and Ramsay, H. (2019). Mental and physical health conditions in people with intellectual disabilities: Comparing local and national data. *British Journal of Learning Disabilities*, 48, pp. 19–27.

Public Health England. (2018). *Learning disabilities: applying All Our Health* [online]. Available at: https://www.gov.uk/government/publications/learning-disability-applying-all-our-health/ learning-disabilities-applying-all-our-health

Roll, A.E. (2018). Health promotion for people with intellectual disabilities – A concept analysis. *Scandinavian Journal of Caring Sciences*, 32, pp. 422–429.

White, A., Sheehan, R., Ding, J., Roberts, C., Magill, N., Keagan-Bull, R., Carter, B., Ruane, M., Xiang, X., Chauhan, U., Tuffrey-Wijne, I. and Strydom, A. (2022). Learning from lives and deaths – People with a learning disability and autistic people (LeDeR). Available at: https://www. kcl.ac.uk/ioppn/assets/fans-dept/leder-main-report-hyperlinked.pdf

12 Health Promotion for Children and Young People

Katriona Cheng

Promoting Children and Young People's Health

In the UK, children and young people are entitled to a programme of universal healthcare provision that aims to ensure optimum health and wellbeing from pre-birth to 19 years of age. In England, this evidence-based universal programme is known as the Healthy Child Programme (Department of Health 2009a, 2009b) and is delivered primarily by midwives, health visitors and school nurses with the support of other healthcare professionals across primary care services. This universal approach provides advice and support on parenting, whilst monitoring the child's growth, health and development. The programme has the flexibility to ensure that children, young people and families with more profound needs receive an enhanced service which is delivered in conjunction with a variety of health and social care professionals. Children and young people can benefit from a huge range of interventions aimed at improving their health status. Key aspects and windows of opportunity for healthcare professionals to promote health to children, young people and their families will be detailed below.

Immunisation

Immunisations or vaccinations are given to stimulate the body to develop active immunity, whereby the individual's own immune system produces protection against an infectious disease (UK Health Security Agency & Department of Health and Social Care 2021). Some protection can be acquired passively, most commonly through the transfer of antibodies from mother to child, though this protection may be temporary.

Our everyday environment exposes humans to numerous infectious agents which leaves young babies particularly vulnerable to infections, so children require several different vaccinations across their childhood to have maximum protection. In the UK, immunisations are routinely given in infancy at 8, 12 and 16 weeks of age, in early childhood after the child's first birthday and when the child is around three and a half years of age. Further immunisations and boosters occur in the early teenage years (UK Health Security Agency 2022).

Oral Health

Maintaining good oral health is crucial to the wellbeing of every child as it has a significant impact on their development, ability to eat, socialise and sleep and their concentration during school or other activities. Over 60,000 school days are missed each year in England

DOI: 10.4324/9781003411321-12

solely due to children having teeth extractions in hospitals (Office for Health Improvement and Disparities 2022a). Public Health England's (2019a) report confirms there is a significantly higher prevalence of dental caries in children who are overweight or very overweight compared to children whose weight is within a healthy range. Dental decay, also known as dental caries, is a disease that affects primary (baby) and permanent (adult) teeth and can occur at any stage of a person's life (Office for Health Improvement and Disparities 2022b). A further Public Health England (2020) report stated that for 5-year-old children in England, the prevalence of having dental decay was 23.4%, ranging from 1.1% in Hastings, East Sussex (an affluent area of the country) to 50.9% in Blackburn with Darwen (a deprived district). Dental decay is associated with deprivation, 13.7% of 5-year-olds living in areas of least deprivation experience dental decay compared to 34.3% for those residing in more deprived areas (Public Health England 2020). However, there are signs that there has been an improvement in dental health in some areas of the country including those in less affluent districts (Public Health England 2020). Adding fluoride to water can reduce dental decay by up to 35% (Iheozor-Ejiofor et al. 2015). Despite this, little progress has been made in rolling this out across the UK as water fluoridation schemes are only provided to approximately 10% of England's population (Office for Health Improvement and Disparities 2022b). Five-year-olds living in areas with a fluoridation scheme or higher fluoride concentrations were less likely to experience dental caries. Similarly, children and young people living in areas with higher fluoride concentrations were over 50% less likely to be admitted to a hospital for tooth extraction compared to those in areas with lower fluoride concentrations (Office for Health Improvement and Disparities 2022b). To have teeth removed due to dental decay, children aged 10 years and under are often admitted to hospital and put under general anaesthetic (Public Health England 2020). This is obviously quite traumatic. Addressing the backlog of tooth extractions for children aged 10 years and under is one of five key areas of focus within the Core20PLUS5 approach to reduce health inequalities (NHS England 2022).

To reduce the number of children who experience dental decay, actions to improve oral health and reduce inequalities are needed, particularly as the majority of dental decay is preventable (Public Health England 2020). This will involve dental services enquiring with parents or carers about supervising teeth brushing, routine oral hygiene and the family diet and providing advice as they will have a significant influence on these daily necessities for the children in their care (National Institute for Health and Care Excellence 2015). Avoiding food and drink with high sugar content before bed is recommended as this is when saliva flow is reduced (Department of Health and Social Care & Office for Health Improvement and Disparities 2021). The starches in sugar take longer to be broken down and get absorbed into the bloodstream which means the sugar lingers in the mouth, attracting harmful bacteria and so producing the acid which dissolves tooth enamel. Dental services should also encourage regular oral check-ups to help children establish effective, sustainable oral hygiene practice (National Institute for Health and Care Excellence 2015).

A wider coordinated approach to improve oral health in environments where children and young people either live or visit often is likely to improve their health and wellbeing. For instance, schools can promote oral health by making water freely available to all students and staff and providing healthy food and drink options in vending machines. Outside of the school environment, some local authorities are evaluating the quality of current food providers near schools and restricting and managing the number of fast food providers to reduce the choice and proximity to students (Public Health England 2014). Through personal, social and health education sessions, students should be provided with the opportunity to learn about what contributes to and maintains a healthy lifestyle including the benefits of healthy eating and dental hygiene.

Promoting well-balanced diets in schools, youth clubs, sports teams, etc. which are low in sugars and high in fruit and vegetables and prioritising consumption of water are strategies to reduce the likelihood of oral diseases (World Health Organization 2022a).

Diet

Closely linked to oral health is the diet we consume. The world is more aware of the evidence linking unhealthy and unbalanced diets to many chronic diseases. Maintaining a healthy weight is crucial throughout pregnancy, childhood and adolescence to reduce the likelihood of health problems later in life. As a result, populations are increasingly choosing foods with fewer calories and lower fat content in order to reap health benefits (Ofori and Hsieh 2007). As the demand for healthier foods increases, food manufacturers are increasingly choosing foods with less calories and lower fat content. A high-sugar diet is a risk factor not only for tooth decay but also for obesity and diabetes (World Health Organization 2022b). Knowing that children especially will not be able to totally avoid sugar, the Department of Health and Social Care & Office for Health Improvement and Disparities (2021) has produced guidance stipulating the maximum daily amounts of added sugar by age (Table 12.1).

In addition, there are free sugars which refer to sugars that naturally occur in honey, syrups, fruit juices and smoothies (Department of Health and Social Care & Office for Health Improvement and Disparities 2021). The Government's recommendation for free sugar consumption within the population should be up to 5% of a person's total energy intake from the age of 2 years onwards (Department of Health and Social Care & Office for Health Improvement and Disparities 2021). A significant amount of children's sugar intake comes from sugar-sweetened beverages, biscuits, cakes, sweets and breakfast cereals (Department of Health and Social Care & Office for Health Improvement and Disparities 2021). Unfortunately, the intake of vegetables and fruit, a healthy alternative, has changed minimally across the population despite the 5 a day campaign that was launched by the Government in 2003. Advice on healthy eating should be encouraged at every opportunity, but the cost and perishable nature of fruit and vegetables may be proving a barrier to some.

The Soft Drinks Industry Levy (SDIL), also known as the sugar tax, came into effect in 2018 to help tackle childhood obesity (Soft Drinks Industry Levy Regulations 2018). It requires soft drink providers to reduce the sugar content of their drinks substantially with levies on drinks containing over 5 g of sugar per 100 ml. The money generated from these fines is being put towards school sports facilities and equipment and providing school breakfast clubs with healthier options with the aim to reduce childhood obesity in the UK (HM Treasury 2018).

Table 12.1 Maximum Daily Recommendations of Added Sugar from Age 4 Years

Age	Recommended Maximum Daily Amount of Added Sugar
4–6 years	5 cubes (19 g)
7–10 years	6 cubes (24 g)
11 years and above	7 cubes (30 g)

Another method to tackle childhood obesity is the National Child Measurement Programme whereby the height and weight measurements of children from state funded schools in reception (aged 4–5 years) and year 6 (aged 10–11 years) are recorded. This equates to over a million children being measured each year and helps the UK government track childhood obesity trends so that policy and interventions can be updated and appropriate actions taken (Local Government Association 2022). Compared to the 2020–2021 academic year, the prevalence of children in reception and year 6 living with obesity has decreased by 4% and 2%, respectively, which is good news, although the prevalence is higher than before the Covid-19 pandemic (NHS Digital 2022). Compared to children who live in the least deprived areas, children living in the most deprived areas are more than twice as likely to live with obesity, indicating these families need the most help to reduce their children's obesity levels (NHS Digital 2022).

Although much more could be done, the food industry has been working with governments to implement strategies to reduce obesity levels. To deter people from purchasing unhealthy snacks, supermarkets have adopted nudging techniques by adjusting their layout to steer people towards healthier choices though less healthy alternatives are still available (Harbers et al. 2020). Supermarket environments will often have fruit and vegetables close to the entrance to encourage subliminal messaging of walking through these aisles and seeing these nutritious foods readily available. Sweets, chocolates, biscuits and alcohol are usually found at the furthest point from the entrance indicating that the purchaser needs to make a conscious effort to get to the furthest part of the shop to obtain these items, passing healthier alternatives on their journey. These foods have also been removed from checkouts so they are out of sight and reach of queuing customers and replaced with healthier alternatives to encourage healthier choices. Research found that between 2016 and 2017, 76% fewer sales of sugary confectionary, chocolate and crisps were recorded in supermarkets with checkout food policies than those without, indicating a significant association between the checkout policies and food purchases (Ejlerskov et al. 2018).

Additionally, product marketing has a significant impact on consumer consumption and influences customers by the product itself, its price, place and promotion (Winkler et al. 2016). Product assortment (the range of products on offer) and availability are crucial to encourage the consumer to consider buying a healthier product. Price is an important factor in choice, particularly for families on lower incomes who may find that healthier food is almost twice the price of unhealthy alternatives and are therefore unwilling to pay more for less food (Kern et al. 2017). The product's location or its place needs to be considered to appeal to the consumers most likely to purchase the item, for example, is it easily found? Are similar products grouped together? Are they at eye level? Or, are certain items only available from specialist retailers and so have to be sought out? Finally, the promotion of the product internally and externally will influence how attractive the product is to a population. This may include having offers or discounts within the store, influencers providing positive reviews on the product and the use of targeted social media or television adverts. All the above aspects could be used by retailers to promote healthier dietary choices.

Schools play a significant role in establishing healthy eating behaviours for pupils. There are several ways that schools can provide and encourage healthy meal options for their pupils and staff. Schools in the UK must adhere to The Requirement for School Food Regulations (2014), which provide strict guidelines for school meals, including the frequency of certain foods on the menu and the availability of condiments and snacks. Reasonable adjustments should be made for those with specific requirements such as for medical, dietary and cultural needs (Department for Education 2021). In the UK, schools are legally required to provide free school lunches to reception, year 1 and year 2 pupils by the Children and Families Act (2014). Additionally, some pupils are eligible for free school meals beyond this age limit if they or their parents are in receipt of certain state benefits. This was estimated to entitle 50,000 more pupils to a free school meal in 2022 (Department for Education 2018).

Schools are also ideally placed to provide education about balanced and nutritious diets in various subjects across the school day, not just within food technology. Healthy eating displays can help students regularly access consistent information across their school environment, and messages with nutritional information can be shared during assemblies, included in communication to parents and within staff and parent meetings (Centres for Disease Control and Prevention 2019). Providing education about nutrition empowers children with knowledge and skills to make healthy eating choices.

Adopting the Make Every Contact Count approach supports individuals to consider interventions to bring about positive and hopefully sustainable change. However, addressing the topic of a person's weight can be sensitive and challenging for practitioners, parents and friends. Public Health England (2019b) suggests using three steps to deliver a brief intervention. These consist of Ask, Advise and Assist. Asking about a person's weight has to be handled delicately to protect the practitioner-patient relationship and not make assumptions. Using a question such as "How would you feel about discussing your weight?" allows the person to consider if this is a topic, they are happy to explore further or if it is something, they don't want to address at this moment. In order to provide advice, the practitioner needs to listen to verbal cues and take note of non-verbal cues, if possible, to see what the patient's initial reaction is to the topic being raised. It involves listening to the priorities for the individual, whether their goals are big and small, and helping the person consider realistic, positive changes they could bring to their lifestyle and that of their children. Finally, enabling people to take control and assisting them to make decisions that best suits them and their lifestyle is an important health promotion concept, even if they try one plan initially but revise this later. This may involve providing further information and/or sign positing to additional services for support.

Physical Activity

In addition to monitoring our dietary intake, physical activity contributes to maintaining a healthy weight. This is particularly important for children and young people as a physical activity contributes to their growth and development. In 2019, Physical Activity Guidelines were published by the UK's Chief Medical Officers emphasising that all age groups can achieve greater health benefits through regular physical activity (Department of Health and Social Care 2019). However, in the 2021–2022 academic year, Sport England (2022) report that only 47.2% of children and young people daily participate in sport and physical activity for the recommended average of 60 minutes or more.

Starting physical activity from infancy and continuing through the first 5 years of life can have a significant impact on short- and long-term health and development outcomes (World Health Organization 2019). Infants can be active through tummy time, rolling, reaching and developing to floor-based play, crawling, pulling to stand and walking for at least 30 minutes a day (Department of Health and Social Care 2019). Once they become a toddler, it is recommended that there should be a minimum of 3 hours of physical activity per day at different intensities and in different environments (dancing, playgrounds, walking, soft play). Children aged 3–4 years should have over an hour of moderate to vigorous physical activity in addition to a further 2 hours of varying physical activities (Department of Health and Social Care 2019). These strengthening activities are important to build healthy bones and develop and maintain strength throughout childhood.

For children and young people aged 5–18 years, each day should include over an hour of moderate to vigorous physical activities to develop muscular fitness, bone strength and motor skills which can be achieved through physical education lessons in school, active travel, after school or weekend activities and sports (Department of Health and Social Care 2019). Sport England's (2022) report found that children and young people's enjoyment of and confidence towards sport and physical activity both dropped by over 4% from pre pandemic levels, with more children reporting less positive attitudes. This suggests there is a need for children and young people to engage in activities they enjoy to reduce periods of inactivity, in the hope that this also has a knock-on positive effect on their mental health and self-esteem. Regular physical activity in children and adolescents is associated with improved academic performance, better mental health, cardiovascular fitness and maintaining a healthy weight (World Health Organization 2022b). Establishing physical activity habits in childhood can prevent or reduce the risk of chronic conditions in adulthood and improve the individual's health and wellbeing with increased benefits for families, communities and the economy by saving significant health and social care resources (Department of Health and Social Care 2019; National Institute for Health and Care Excellence 2009).

Physical activity guidelines for children vary according to their age. Those under five years of age should partake in three hours of physical activity each day, and children and young people between 5 and 18 years should do 60 minutes of activity daily (NHS UK 2022). However, it is widely recognised that there is still a significant gap in activity levels between genders in the UK. This starts in late adolescence whereby almost two thirds (64%) of girls aged 16–17 years will have quit sport (Hollingsworth 2022). Whilst 78% of girls acknowledge that having an active lifestyle is important by the age of 14–16 years, only 28% expressed enjoyment from participating in physical activity (Women In Sport 2019).

Activity

- Can you think of some barriers specific to teenage girls which dissuade them from sport and exercise?
- What interventions or approaches might help encourage teenage girls to engage in more physical activity?
- Who could be involved and what resources would be needed to develop and initiate these activities?

One campaign example is This Girl Can which was launched in 2015 with the aim to increase and celebrate physical movement of all women and girls nationwide (Sport England 2021). The campaign also recognised that women were afraid of being judged by others predominantly about their appearance during exercise and focused on empowering women with the confidence to exercise despite these fears. The results the campaign achieved would suggest that more women developed confidence which led to increased activity to overcome these barriers. After the first phase of the campaign in 2015, 250,000 more women were active or played sport once a week every week (Sport England 2021). Up until the Covid-19 pandemic, large numbers of women had taken action as a direct result of the campaign and more women participated in sport routinely (Sport England 2021). This progress was hindered by the disruption to physical activity behaviour during the Covid-19 pandemic (Sport England 2021).

Relationships and Sexual Health

As children become adolescents, they require education and support to foster healthy relationships, sexuality and sex which all contribute to their health and wellbeing in addition to information to help assess and minimise risks. During this transition through puberty and increasing independence, teenagers are likely to experience peer pressure and may be coerced into risky sexual health behaviour, increasing to the likelihood of teenage pregnancy and sexually transmitted diseases (Schutt-Aine and Maddaleno 2003). The reduction in teenage pregnancy has been a success story within public health; once the UK had one of the highest rates in Europe. Teenage conception rates in 2007 for girls aged 15–17 years were 41.6 conceptions per 1,000 women in England and Wales, but has declined significantly and in 2020 reached a record low of 13.1 conceptions per 1,000 women (Office for National Statistics 2020). The rate has also decreased for girls under 16 years of age from 2.5 conceptions per 1,000 women in 2019 to 2.1 in 2020 (Office for National Statistics 2020).

Addressing teenage sexual health is complex due to societal views towards this age group and the hormonal and behaviour changes puberty brings. Previously, there has been a strong focus towards the negative outcomes of sexual behaviour; however, now there is a greater shift towards a positive approach, viewing diversity, sexuality and sex as a valid part of holistic wellbeing and its contributions to health and happiness (Bailey et al. 2015; Helbekkmo et al. 2021). In 2020, relationship and sex education was made statutory in all secondary schools in England, along with relationship education in primary schools and health education across both school settings (Public Health England 2018). Sex education that is inclusive of all sexualities and cultures helps young people develop social and emotional skills along with the appreciation of sexual diversities and a greater awareness of intimate partner violence. Content should be tailored to the relevant age group and include human biology, healthy, safe and enjoyable relationships initially, building to include mental health, child sexual abuse and exploitation, both to empower children and young people and ensure that they take these values and healthy behaviours into adulthood (Public Health England 2018). However, there is a wide variation in the provision of sex and relationships education with some schools providing lots of information and support and others providing minimal information, skills and resources which hinders young people from learning about safe relationships and sex (Bailey et al. 2015). Additionally, children are allowed to be withdrawn from planned sex education by their parents, reducing their exposure to safe and healthy relationships and sex education further.

Professional external educators who can provide different perspectives are more effective than teachers and can help students feel at ease (Helbekkmo et al. 2021). Equally, some students prefer to discuss topics with their teachers if they have a pre-existing relationship and feel safe talking about sensitive issues (Helbekkmo et al. 2021). Interactive digital interventions for sexual health can be useful. Whilst internet access is widely available to almost all children through their home or school, young people may not have open access to sexual health content due to sharing devices at home, in school or with filters to prevent young people from accessing further inappropriate content (Bailey et al. 2015). To broaden their reach, the interactive digital interventions could be linked with relevant partner agencies such as sexually transmitted infection clinics, trusted websites linked to sex education and potentially social networking platforms (Bailey et al. 2015). Face-to-face consultations and regular engagement will also provide advice, monitoring of progress and support to maintain healthy sexual health. Delivery through mixed methods is more likely to provide access to the target population (Bailey et al. 2015).

Summary

In the UK, over 9 million pupils attended education in the 2021–2022 academic year from nursery to secondary school (Office for National Statistics 2022). Whilst at school, children and young people develop lifelong behaviours and attitudes towards their health, and hence health promotion is crucial in this environment to encourage pupils to adopt these and recognise the impact on their entire lives. Staff, the pupils' families and the wider community are also likely to benefit from these health promotion messages directly and indirectly demonstrating the ripple effect these messages can have beyond the individual pupils.

Addressing inequalities, reducing deprivation levels and improving social determinants of health with an emphasis on children, young people and their families need to be a key focus for policy makers when creating and implementing policies and guidelines (Kossarova et al. 2017). It is recognised that emergency care is prioritised and with limited resources many prevention and early intervention services are experiencing significant pressure, despite the fact that hospital admissions could be reduced with the provision of and early access to high quality children's health services (Kossarova et al. 2017). Services need to be provided at the universal population level for all children and families along with targeted services for children with developing needs or at risk of poorer outcomes and specialist services for children and families where specialist intervention is required.

References

Bailey, J., Mann, S., Wayal, S., Hunter, R., Free, C., Abraham, C. and Murray, E. (2015). Sexual health promotion for young people delivered via digital media: A scoping review. *Public Health Research*, 3(13). https://www.journalslibrary.nihr.ac.uk/phr/phr03130/#/full-report
Centres for Disease Control and Prevention. (2019). *Opportunities for nutrition education in US schools.* https://www.cdc.gov/healthyschools/nutrition/pdf/308155-A_FS_SchoolNutritionEd-508.pdf
Children and Families Act. (2014). *Children and Families Act 2014.* (c.6). Great Britain, London: The Stationary Office. https://www.legislation.gov.uk/ukpga/2014/6/contents/enacted
Department for Education. (2018). *Free school meals.* https://assets.publishing.service.gov.uk/government/uploads/system/uploads/attachment_data/file/700139/Free_school_meals_guidance_Apr18.pdf
Department for Education. (2021). *School food in England.* https://www.gov.uk/government/publications/standards-for-school-food-in-england/school-food-in-england
Department of Health. (2009a). *Healthy Child Programme: From 5-19 years old.* https://assets.publishing.service.gov.uk/government/uploads/system/uploads/attachment_data/file/492086/HCP_5_to_19.pdf
Department of Health. (2009b). *Healthy Child Programme: Pregnancy and the first five years of life.* https://assets.publishing.service.gov.uk/government/uploads/system/uploads/attachment_data/file/167998/Health_Child_Programme.pdf
Department of Health and Social Care. (2019). *UK Chief Medical Officers' Physical Activity Guidelines.* chrome-extension://efaidnbmnnnibpcajpcglclefindmkaj/https://assets.publishing.service.gov.uk/government/uploads/system/uploads/attachment_data/file/832868/uk-chief-medical-officers-physical-activity-guidelines.pdf
Department of Health and Social Care & Office for Health Improvement and Disparities. (2021). *Healthier eating.* https://www.gov.uk/government/publications/delivering-better-oral-health-an-evidence-based-toolkit-for-prevention/chapter-10-healthier-eating

Ejlerskov, K., Sharp, S., Stead, M., Adamson, A., White, M. and Adams, J. (2018). Supermarket policies on less-healthy food at checkouts: Natural experimental evaluation using interrupted time series analyses of purchases. *Public Library of Science Medicine*, 15(12). https://pubmed.ncbi.nlm.nih.gov/30562349/

Harbers, M., Beulens, J., Rutters, F., de Boer, F., Gillebart, M., Sluijs, I. and van der Schouw, Y. (2020). The effects of nudges of purchases, food choice and energy intake or content of purchases in real-life food purchasing environments: A systematic review and evidence synthesis. *Nutrition Journal*, 19, 1–27. https://nutritionj.biomedcentral.com/articles/10.1186/s12937-020-00623-y#citeas

Helbekkmo, E., Tempero, H.T., Sollesnes, R. and Langeland, E. (2021). 'We expected more about sex in the sex week' - a qualitative study about students' experiences with a sexual health education programme, from a health-promotion perspective. *International Journal of Qualitative Studies on Health and Well-Being*, 16(1). https://doi.org/10.1080/17482631.2021.1963035

HM Treasury. (2018). *Soft Drinks Industry Levy comes into effect.* https://www.gov.uk/government/news/soft-drinks-industry-levy-comes-into-effect

Hollingsworth, T. (2022). *We need to keep pushing.* Sport England. https://www.sportengland.org/blogs/we-need-keep-pushing#:~:text=And%20the%20gender%20gap%20starts,social%20rewards%20of%20getting%20active.

Iheozor-Ejiofor, Z., Worthington, H., Walsh, T., O'Malley, L., Clarkson, J., Macey, R., Alam, R., Tugwell, P., Welch, V. and Glenny, A.-M. (2015). Water fluoridation for the prevention of dental caries. *Cochrane Database of Systematic Reviews*, 6. https://doi.org/10.1002/14651858.CD010856.pub2

Kern, D., Auchnicloss, A., Stehr, M., Diez Roux, A., Moore, L., Kanter, G. and Robinson, L. (2017). Neighbourhood prices of healthier and unhealthier foods and associations with diet quality: Evidence from the multi-ethnic study of atherosclerosis. *International Journal of Environmental Research and Public Health*, 14(11). https://www.ncbi.nlm.nih.gov/pmc/articles/PMC5708033/pdf/ijerph-14-01394.pdf

Kossarova, L., Cheung, R., Hargreaves, D. and Keeble, E. (2017). *Admissions of inequality: Emergency hospital use for children and young people.* https://www.nuffieldtrust.org.uk/files/2017-12/nt-admissions-of-inequality-web.pdf

Local Government Association. (2022). *Must know: Healthy weight.* https://www.local.gov.uk/publications/must-know-healthy-weight#:~:text=The%20NCMP%20was%20established%20in,%2C%20including%20academies%2C%20in%20England

National Institute for Health and Care Excellence. (2009). *Physical activity for children and young people.* https://www.nice.org.uk/guidance/ph17/resources/physical-activity-for-children-and-young-people-pdf-1996181580229

National Institute for Health and Care Excellence. (2015). *Oral health promotion: General dental practice.* https://www.nice.org.uk/guidance/ng30/resources/oral-health-promotion-general-dental-practice-pdf-1837385644741

NHS Digital. (2022). *National Child Measurement Programme, England, 2021/22 school year.* https://digital.nhs.uk/data-and-information/publications/statistical/national-child-measurement-programme/2021-22-school-year

NHS England. (2022). *Core20PLUS5 - An approach to reducing health inequalities for children and young people.* https://www.england.nhs.uk/about/equality/equality-hub/national-healthcare-inequalities-improvement-programme/core20plus5/core20plus5-cyp/

NHS UK. (2022). *Physical activity guidelines for children and young people.* https://www.nhs.uk/live-well/exercise/exercise-guidelines/physical-activity-guidelines-children-and-young-people/

Office for Health Improvement and Disparities. (2022a). *Child oral health: Applying all our health.* https://www.gov.uk/government/publications/child-oral-health-applying-all-our-health/child-oral-health-applying-all-our-health

Office for Health Improvement and Disparities. (2022b). *Water fluoridation - Health monitoring report for England 2022.* https://assets.publishing.service.gov.uk/government/uploads/system/uploads/attachment_data/file/1060471/water-fluoridation-health-monitoring-report-2022.pdf

Office for National Statistics. (2020, April). *Conceptions in England and Wales: 2020.* https://www. ons.gov.uk/peoplepopulationandcommunity/birthsdeathsandmarriages/conceptionandfertilityrates/ bulletins/conceptionstatistics/2020

Office for National Statistics. (2022, June). *Academic year 2021/22: Schools pupils and their characteristics.* https://explore-education-statistics.service.gov.uk/find-statistics/school-pupils-and-their-characteristics

Ofori, J.A. and Hsieh, Y.-H.P. (2007). Innovations in food technology for health. *Asia Pacific Journal of Clinical Nutrition,* 16, pp. 65–73. https://apjcn.nhri.org.tw/server/APJCN/16%20Suppl%201/65.pdf

Public Health England. (2014). *Local authorities improving oral health: Commissioning better oral health for children and young people.* https://assets.publishing.service.gov.uk/government/uploads/ system/uploads/attachment_data/file/321503/CBOHMaindocumentJUNE2014.pdf

Public Health England. (2018). *Teenage pregnancy prevention framework.* https://assets.publishing. service.gov.uk/government/uploads/system/uploads/attachment_data/file/836597/Teenage_ Pregnancy_Prevention_Framework.pdf

Public Health England. (2019a). *The relationship between dental caries and body mass index: Child level analysis.* https://assets.publishing.service.gov.uk/government/uploads/system/uploads/ attachment_data/file/844121/BMI_dental_caries.pdf

Public Health England. (2019b). *A healthier weight - Birth to age four.* https://khub.net/web/phe-national/ public-library/-/document_library/v2WsRK3ZlEig/view_file/262823635?_com_liferay_document_ library_web_portlet_DLPortlet_INSTANCE_v2WsRK3ZlEig_redirect=https%3A%2F%2Fkhub. net%3A443%2Fweb%2Fphe-national%2Fpublic-library%2F-%2Fdocument_library%2 Fv2WsRK3ZlEig%2Fview%2F262823140%3F_com_liferay_document_library_web_port let_DLPortlet_INSTANCE_v2WsRK3ZlEig_redirect%3Dhttps%253A%252F%252Fkhub. net%253A443%252Fweb%252Fphe-national%252Fpublic-library%252F-%252Fdocument_libr ary%252Fv2WsRK3ZlEig%252Fview%252F175783630

Public Health England. (2020). *National Dental Epidemiology Programme for England: Oral health survey of 5 year olds 2019.* https://assets.publishing.service.gov.uk/government/uploads/system/ uploads/attachment_data/file/873492/NDEP_for_England_OH_Survey_5yr_2019_v1.0.pdf

Schutt-Aine, J. and Maddaleno, M. (2003). *Sexual health and development of adolescents and youth in the Americas: Program and policy implications.* https://www1.paho.org/English/HPP/HPF/ ADOL/SRH.pdf

Soft Drinks Industry Levy Regulations. (2018). *Soft Drinks Industry Levy Regulations 2018* (No. 41). Great Britain, London: The Stationary Office. https://www.legislation.gov.uk/uksi/2018/41/ contents/made

Sport England. (2021). *This girl can campaign summary.* https://sportengland-production-files.s3.eu-west-2.amazonaws.com/s3fs-public/2022-05/TGC%20Campaign%20summary%202021_0.pdf? VersionId=8j5WaQWXjRZy95JkiyT8s_8efCG.8llF

Sport England. (2022). *Active Lives Children and Young People Survey Academic Year 2021-22.* https://sportengland-production-files.s3.eu-west-2.amazonaws.com/s3fs-public/2022-12/ Active%20Lives%20Children%20and%20Young%20People%20Survey%20Academic%20 Year%202021-22%20Report.pdf?VersionId=R5_hmJHw5M4yKFsewm2vGDMRGHWW7q3E

The Requirement for School Food Regulations. (2014). *The Requirement for School Food Regulations 2014* (No. 1603). Great Britain, London: The Stationary Office https://www.legislation.gov. uk/uksi/2014/1603/contents/made

UK Health Security Agency. (2022, February). *The routine immunisation schedule.* https://assets. publishing.service.gov.uk/government/uploads/system/uploads/attachment_data/file/1055877/ UKHSA-12155-routine-complete-immunisation-schedule_Feb2022.pdf

UK Health Security Agency & Department of Health and Social Care. (2021). Immunity and how vaccines work: The green book, in *The Green Book: Immunisation against infectious disease.* https://assets.publishing.service.gov.uk/government/uploads/system/uploads/attachment_data/ file/949797/Greenbook_chapter_1_Jan21.pdf

Winkler, L., Christensen, U., Glümer, C., Bloch, P., Mikkelsen, B., Wansink, B. and Toft, U. (2016). Substituting sugar confectionary with fruit and healthy snacks at checkout - A win-win strategy for consumers and food stores? A study on consumer attitudes and sales effects of a healthy supermarket intervention. *BMC Public Health*, 16. https://bmcpublichealth.biomedcentral.com/articles/10.1186/s12889-016-3849-4

Women In Sport. (2019). *Reframing sport for teenage girls: Building strong foundations for their futures*. https://www.gmmoving.co.uk/media/2544/women-in-sport-teenage-girls-dropping-out-of-sport-and-pa.pdf

World Health Organization. (2019). *Guidelines on physical activity, sedentary behaviour and sleep for children under 5 years of age*. https://www.who.int/publications/i/item/9789241550536

World Health Organization. (2022a). *Oral health*. https://www.who.int/news-room/fact-sheets/detail/oral-health

World Health Organization. (2022b). *Physical activity*. https://www.who.int/news-room/fact-sheets/detail/physical-activity

13 Physical Activity Promotion

Michelle Turner

Introduction and Key Concepts

Physical activity levels in the United Kingdom (UK) have declined over the past decades. Currently, adults are at least 20% less active than they were in the 1960s, and estimates suggest that by 2030 this will increase to 35% (Ng and Popkin 2012). Studies in the UK looked at physical activity levels and risk of non-communicable diseases and found an increased risk between 19% and 66% of developing coronary heart disease, type 2 diabetes and breast and colon cancers for those leading inactive lives (Lee et al. 2012). Inactivity shortens life expectancy and contributes to one in six deaths, which is comparable with the effects of smoking (Wen and Wu 2012). The World Health Organization (WHO 2009) places physical inactivity as the fourth biggest risk factor for the development of non-communicable diseases in high income countries.

Definition of Activity

Physical activity is defined as 'any bodily movement produced by skeletal muscles that requires energy expenditure. It takes many forms, occurs in many settings, and has many purposes (daily activity, active recreation, and sport)' (Department of Health and Social Care [DHSC] 2019, p. 14). Different types of activity are required for individual health needs and to achieve different benefits. Health enhancing physical activity includes multiple types of activity, including, cardiovascular, muscle and bone strengthening, balance training and breaking up periods of sedentary time (DHSC 2019).

Benefits of Physical Activity – Our Past and Present

Researchers such as Eaton, Konner and Shostak. (1988) have suggested that hunter gatherers, in Palaeolithic times, followed a rhythm of intense activity, followed by rest periods and more moderate activity. This level of physical activity is still required by mankind today and is reflected in the UK guidelines for adults, which recommend 150 minutes of moderate intensity activity or 75 minutes of vigorous activity a week (DHSC 2019). There's been no biological change in humans in 50,000 years and yet present-day activity levels are so vastly different from our ancestors. Gould (2000) suggests that this mismatch between western lifestyles and genetics may be the main cause for diseases of civilisation. There is a proven correlation between those living active lives and the reduced risk of disease, improved mental health and increased vitality and longevity. Regular physical activity improves cognitive function and reduces the risk of dementia, reduces the risk of certain cancers and disease

DOI: 10.4324/9781003411321-13

progression for conditions such as osteoarthritis, hypertension and type 2 diabetes, reduces excessive weight gain in adults, children and pregnant women, reduces anxiety levels and improves sleep (Physical Activity Guidelines Committee [PAG] 2018). Harvard researchers are exploring evolutionary and biomedical evidence between activity levels in later life and the inflammatory processes leading to disease (Lieberman et al. 2021). Wider benefits include improving connections to our community and nature, increasing happiness and adding purpose to life (Sports England 2017).

The Scale of the Problem

Health surveys undertaken in the UK show that only 58–64% of adults achieve the physical activity levels required for good health (DHSC 2019). The WHO states that worldwide, approximately one in four adults, and three in four, 11–17-year-olds, do not meet the global recommendations for physical activity and in some countries, inactivity levels are as high as 70% (WHO 2018). In the UK, approximately one-third of men's and half of women's health will be harmed by a lack of physical activity (Public Health England [PHE] 2014). Activity levels for people who develop more than one chronic condition show a further decline, with only 31% of people living with three impairments achieving the recommended guidelines (Sports England 2021).

The Need for Government Strategy

The reasons for inactivity are varied and complex and Sallis et al. (2021) conclude the necessity for government departments to provide the infrastructure alongside equitable access and opportunities to enable populations to increase activity. The UK government following from the Marmot review (2010) has again stated that addressing inequalities is high on their agenda as areas of deprivation have the highest inactivity levels (DHSC 2019). The 'Gear change, A bold vision for walking and cycling' document sets out an ambition to transform the role cycling and walking have in our transport system in an effort to increase activity (Department for Transport [DfT] 2016). A good example of how legislation supports the public to make lifestyle changes is a recent change to the UK Highway code. This change gives a greater priority to pedestrians and cyclists over cars at junctions and crossings (Government UK 2022). A reduction in car use and, therefore, emissions would also result in the benefit of cleaner air and a step towards addressing climate change. The ability to make lifestyle changes goes hand in hand with legislation to support and enable the population.

UK Physical Activity Guidelines

In 2011, the UK's Chief Medical Officer (CMO) developed the first physical activity guidance (DHSC 2011). After a review of the evidence surrounding physical activity, new guidelines were developed to cover the life course, including for ante and postnatal women and for people of all ages living with a disability (DHSC 2019, 2022). The new guidance shone a light on the damaging effect sedentary lives have on our health and the need for strength and balance activities in addition to aerobic activity. Whilst the recommended amount of activity for good health remains unchanged, evidence confirms that we gain from even small amounts of movement, and just two minutes of physical activity per day has physical and physiological benefits (Dunstan et al. 2012). There is a multifaceted dose-response curve between inactive people and increased movement, and those most inactive stand to gain the most as they begin to move more (PHE 2018). It is important to emphasise that everyone has their own starting point, and there is a wide variety of options available, whether that is joining a walking group, a park run or dancing at home, promoting 'movement snacking' in whatever way works for the individual (MIND 2022).

The Role of the Healthcare Professional

There is evidence to suggest one in four people would be more active if spoken to by a family doctor or nurse (PHE 2014). Lobelo and Quevedo (2016) discuss that healthcare professionals who lead active lives are more likely to discuss physical activity with patients. Conversely, in 2017, a study found only 25% of family doctors regularly discussed the benefits of activity (Chatterjee et al. 2017). It appears that healthcare professionals can be fearful of encouraging people to be active due to fear of harm whilst the opposite is a reality (Reid et al. 2022). The 'Moving health care professionals programme' in England delivers training to healthcare professionals, helping them in their critical role of helping others to move more (Sports England 2022).

Focus on Physical Activity for Specific Groups

The Overweight or Obese

Increasing physical activity to aid a weight loss programme is proven to be positive (PAG 2018) but the evidence that it contributes considerably to weight loss is not conclusive (Cox 2017). However, Kettle et al. (2022) studied people who were overweight and found a sustained 1 kg weight loss for those increasing activity. Whilst this is a modest loss, it is still significant as it aligns to health improvements. Recent studies indicate that if activity levels are high, irrelevant of weight status, there is an association with decreased mortality and it is hypothesised that this is due to the disruption within the multiple metabolic pathways (Tarp et al. 2021). Lee et al. (2012) also found that achieving higher physical activity levels reduced the probability of mortality from breast cancer. In fact, higher activity levels provided mitigations to overweight women putting their mortality risk comparable to inactive women of a healthy weight status.

Primary Prevention for Children and Young People

The need for our next generations to be active is one of the key aims of Public Health (DHSC 2019). There is evidence of a connection between physical activity levels in childhood continuing into adult life, and hence the need to establish healthy habits for life is an important preventive strategy (Telama et al. 2014). Global evidence suggests girls are less active than boys and this continues across the life course (Telama et al. 2014). Green (2007) advocates to successfully increase activity levels in childhood, a more option-based, recreational approach to physical education (PE) in school rather than a competitive sport is needed.

Interview with a Physical Education (PE) Lead at a UK Primary School

How do you implement the government recommended target of achieving 30 minutes of activity into the school day?

'We have active playtimes with lots of interesting resources and our pupil champions and trained supervisors lead activity sessions. Our PE lessons include formal sports, swimming lessons and pupil led sessions'.

What do you want the children to learn from PE lessons?

'We have extended one of our PE lessons to one hour. The pupils get used to the feel of their heart beating faster and breathing heavier as they exercise for longer. I want them to explore their own capabilities and increase both fitness and confidence. I aim that every child leaves school with the skills and the love of at least one activity or sport that will allow them to keep active for life. The skills to be active are as important as those to read and write'.

What helps you to succeed?

'Being an active person'.

'A holistic school approach to our children's development which includes health and well-being'.

'Engaging with support services, our excellent School games organisers who help us to be an Active school'.

Physical Activity to Combat Depression and Inflammatory Disease

There is strong evidence that physical activity improves mood and quality of sleep and decreases fatigue leading to an antidepressant effect (Schuch et al. 2016). One model of mental health recovery 'CHIME' emphasises connectedness, hope, identity, meaning in life and empowerment (Leamy et al. 2011). Being physically active can help to achieve these important human needs. Providing green and open spaces to enable outdoor activity can help people benefit from both nature and activity for their mental health (DfT 2016).

Evidence suggests 50% of all deaths are somewhat attributable to inflammation, for example, type 2 diabetes and heart disease (Furman et al. 2019). Physical activity plays a role in reducing inflammation. There are many physiological mechanisms that contribute to this, building muscle is one example. Muscle is the most metabolically active tissue in the body and there is a subsequent reduction of systemic inflammation with increased muscle movements (Bay and Pedersen 2020).

Tertiary Prevention for Those in Hospital

The end 'PJ paralysis' concept encourages patients in the hospital to get up, dressed and move, aiming to prevent complications of being immobile such as blood clots (Meesters et al. 2019). This can shift the patients' perceptions from the sick role to one of recovery. In the UK, 'Active hospital' toolkits aim to incorporate movement into recovery (Moving Medicines 2022).

Barriers to Physical Activity

Risks Versus Benefits

Fear of injury or exacerbating symptoms is a barrier to increasing activity (Richmond Charities 2016). A consensus statement was developed to address this and concluded that the benefits of physical activity outweigh the risks for people living with long-term health conditions (Reid et al. 2022). Infographics were designed to provide health professionals with evidenced-based reference guides, helping them to address the most cited barriers. Consistent messaging is important for people to build trust to follow the advice. Experience of mixed messaging during the Covid-19 pandemic highlights this (Benham et al. 2021). The provision of the consensus statement aims to assist with consistent messaging around physical activity for those living with a disability.

Covid-19

Mitigations to keep us safe and control the Covid-19 virus such as lockdowns, school closures, working from home and shielding increased sedentary time and changed normal activity levels. Initially, there was positive news including a surge in sign up to the UK National Health Service Couch to 5 km app, with downloads rocketing by 92% (National Health Service [NHS] 2021). However, Sports England (2021) indicated that 100,000 (2.3%) children and young people were less active in 2021, and the impact was higher in boys than girls. Sports England (2021) surmises the biggest reduction in activity levels was found in the most disadvantaged populations, such as the unemployed, those living with a disability and ethnic communities. The UK CMO guidelines recommend achieving above 7000 steps a day for better immune function (Tudor-Locke et al. 2011). A study in South Korea (Cho et al. 2021) showed an association between those achieving higher levels of activity and a reduction in infection rates and mortality from Covid-19. These studies highlight the benefit physical activity plays in reducing the impact of communicable diseases on individuals.

Activity

Research physical activity opportunities, initiatives and resources locally and nationally.
Refer to the 'Moving Medicines' website (available at https://movingmedicine. ac.uk) and make a crib sheet of key sentences you can use to address the barriers and fears of becoming more active than you can use with your client group.

Conclusion

Sir Chris Whitty when he was the UK's Chief Medical Officer stated, 'There is no situation, there is no age and no condition where exercise is not a good thing' (British Broadcasting Corporation [BBC] 2020). There is significant worldwide research and policy supporting increasing physical activity levels in order to optimise health across the life course. Adequate infrastructure and equitable opportunity are needed to enable people to lead active lives. Increasing physical activity levels has the potential to improve the health of the nations.

Key Messages

- Achieving recommended activity levels improves mental and physical health outcomes.
- By leading an active life, we can inspire friends, family and our communities to be active too, 'it's never too late to start' (DHSC 2019).
- It is safe for most people to move more.
- Risk of adverse events is low but that is not how people feel; sharing the available resources and evidence will help reduce this fear.
- People need to have an individual plan from their starting point and help to build confidence.

- We need government support to provide the infrastructure and equitable opportunities to achieve the recommended levels of activity for good health.
- 'Every minute counts, Some is good, more is better' (DHSC 2019, p. 44).

References

Bay, M.L. and Pedersen, B.K. (2020). Muscle-organ crosstalk: Focus on immunometabolism. *Frontiers in Physiology*, 11, 567881. https://doi.org/10.3389/fphys.2020.567881

Benham, J.L., Lang, R., Burns, K., MacKean, G., Le´veille´, T., McCormack, B., Sheikh, H., Fullerton, M., Tang, T., Boucher, Constantinescu, C., Mourali, M., Oxoby, J. and Manns, R., M. and Marshall, M. (2021). Attitudes, current behaviours and barriers to public health measures that reduce COVID-19 transmission: A qualitative study to inform public health messaging. *PLoS ONE*, 16(2), e0246941. https://doi.org/10.1371/journal.pone.0246941

British Broadcasting Corporation (BBC). (2020). *Coronavirus stay fit to fight the virus, says medic.* Available at: https://www.bbc.co.uk/news/uk-52076856

Chatterjee, R., Chapman, T., Brannan, M.G. and Varney, J. (2017). GPs' knowledge, use, and confidence in national physical activity and health guidelines and tools: A questionnaire-based survey of general practice in England. *The British Journal of General Practice: The Journal of the Royal College of General Practitioners*, 67(663), pp. e668–e675. https://doi.org/10.3399/bjgp17X692513

Cho, D.H., Lee, S.J., Jae, S.Y., Kim, W.J., Ha, S.J., Gwon, J.G., Choi, J., Kim, D.W. and Kim, J.Y. (2021). Physical activity and the risk of COVID-19 infection and mortality: A nationwide population-based case-control study. *Journal of Clinical Medicine*, 10(7), p. 1539. https://doi.org/10.3390/jcm10071539.

Cox, C.E. (2017). Role of physical activity for weight loss and weight maintenance. *Diabetes Spectrum: A Publication of the American Diabetes Association*, 30(3), pp. 157–160. https://doi.org/10.2337/ds17-0013.

Department for Transport (DfT). (2016). *Gear change. A bold vision for cycling and walking.* London. Available at: https://assets.publishing.service.gov.uk/government/uploads/system/uploads/attachment_data/file/904146/gear-change-a-bold-vision-for-cycling-and-walking.pdf

Department of Health and Social Care (DHSC). (2011). *Start active, stay active report.* Available at: https://www.gov.uk/government/publications/start-active-stay-active-a-report-on-physical-activity-from-the-four-home-countries-chief-medical-officers

Department of Health and Social Care (DHSC). (2019). *UK Chief Medical Officer's physical activity guidelines.* Available at: https://www.gov.uk/government/publications/physical-activity-guidelines-uk-chief-medical-officers-report

Department of Health and Social Care (DHSC). (2022). *UK Chief Medical Officer guidelines on physical activity for disabled children and disabled young people methodology.* Available at: https://www.gov.uk/government/publications/physical-activity-guidelines-disabled-children-and-disabled-young-people

Dunstan, D.W., Kingwell, B.A., Larsen, R., Healy, G.N., Cerin, E., Hamilton, M.T., Shaw, J.E., Bertovic, D.A., Zimmet, P.Z., Salmon, J. and Owen, N. (2012). Breaking up prolonged sitting reduces postprandial glucose and insulin responses. *Diabetes Care* 35(5), pp. 976–983. https://doi.org/10.2337/dc11-1931.

Eaton, M., Konner, M. and Shostak, M. (1988). Stone agers in the fast lane: Chronic degenerative disease evolutionary perspective. *The American Journal of Medicine* (84). Available at: https://www.academia.edu/19090198/Eaton_Konner_Shostak_1988_Stone_agers_in_the_fast_lane_chronic_degenerative_diseases_in_evolutionary_perspective

Furman, D., Campisi, J., Verdin, E., Carrera-Bastos, P., Targ, S., Franceschi, C., Ferrucci, L., Gilroy, D., Fasano, G., Miller, Miller, A., Mantovani, A., Weyand, C., Barzilai, N., Goronzy, J., Rando, T., Effros, R., Lucia, L., Kleinstreuer, N. and Slavich, G. (2019). Chronic inflammation in the etiology of disease across the life span. *Natural Medicine* 25, pp. 1822–1832. https://doi.org/10.1038/s41591-019-0675-0.

Gould, S.J. (2000). The Spice of Life Leader to Leader. 15:14–19. Available at: https://emilkirkegaard.dk/en/wp-content/uploads/SJ-Gould-leader-to-leader-pages.pdf

Government UK. (2022). *The Highway code: 8 changes you need to know by January 29th 2022*. Available at: https://www.gov.uk/government/news/the-highway-code-8-changes-you-need-to-know-from-29-january-2022

Green, K. (2007). *Physical education, lifelong participation and "the couch potato society"*. https://doi.org/10.1080/1740898042000208133.

Kettle, V.E., Madigan, C.D., Coombe, A., Graham, H., Thomas, J.J.C., Chalkley, A.E. and Daley, A. (2022). Effectiveness of physical activity interventions delivered or prompted by health professionals in primary care settings: Systematic review and meta-analysis of randomised controlled trials *British Medical Journal*, 376, e068465. https://doi.org/10.1136/bmj-2021-068465.

Leamy, M., Bird, V., Le Boutillier, C., Williams, J. and Slade, M. (2011). Conceptual framework for personal recovery in mental health: Systematic review and narrative synthesis. *The British Journal of Psychiatry: the Journal of Mental Science*, 199(6), pp. 445–452. https://doi.org/10.1192/bjp.bp.110.083733.

Lee, I.M., Shiroma, E.J., Lobelo, F., Puska, P., Blair, S.N. and Katzmarzyk, P.T. (2012). Lancet physical activity series working group. Effect of physical inactivity on major non-communicable diseases worldwide: An Analysis of burden of disease and life expectancy. *Lancet*, 380(9838), pp. 219–229. https://doi.org/10.1016/S0140-6736(12)61031-9. PMID: 22818936; PMCID: PMC3645500.

Lieberman, D.E., Kistner, T.M., Richard, D., Lee, I.M. and Baggish, A.L. (2021). The active grandparent hypothesis: Physical activity and the evolution of extended human healthspans and lifespans. *Proceedings of the National Academy of Sciences of the United States of America*, 118(50), e2107621118. https://doi.org/10.1073/pnas.2107621118.

Lobelo, F. and de Quevedo, I.G. (2016). The evidence in support of physicians and health care providers as physical activity role models. *American Journal of Lifestyle Medicine*, 10(1), pp. 36–52. https://doi.org/10.1177/1559827613520120.

Meesters, J., Conijn, D., Vermeulen, H.M. and Vlieland, T. (2019). Physical activity during hospitalization: Activities and preferences of adults versus older adults. *Physiotherapy Theory and Practice*, 35(10), pp. 975–985. https://doi.org/10.1080/09593985.2018.1460429. Epub April 16, 2018. PMID: 29658797.

MIND. (2022). *We are undefeatable*. Available at: https://www.mind.org.uk/about-us/our-policy-work/sport-physical-activity-and-mental-health/we-are-undefeatable/

Moving Medicines. (2022). *Active hospital toolkit*. Available at: https://movingmedicine.ac.uk/active-hospitals/

National Health Service (NHS). (2021). *Couch to 5 k*. Available at: https://www.england.nhs.uk/2020/07/around-one-million-downloads-of-fitness-app-during-lockdown-as-people-stay-fit/

Ng, S.W. and Popkin, B.M. (2012). Time use and physical activity: A shift away from movement across the globe. *Obesity Reviews: An Official Journal of the International Association for the Study of Obesity*, 13(8), pp. 659–680. https://doi.org/10.1111/j.1467-789X.2011.00982.x

Physical Activity Guidelines Committee (PAG). (2018). *Advisory Committee report*. Available at: https://health.gov/paguidelines/second-edition/report/pdf/PAG_Advisory_Committee_Report.pdf

Public Health England (PHE). (2014). *Everybody active every day. An evidenced approach to physical activity*. Available at: https://assets.publishing.service.gov.uk/government/uploads/system/uploads/attachment_data/file/374914/Framework_13.pdf

Public Health England (PHE). (2018). *Physical activity for general health benefits in disabled adults: Summary of a rapid evidence review for the UK Chief Medical Officers' update of the physical activity guidelines*. Available at: https://assets.publishing.service.gov.uk/government/uploads/system/uploads/attachment_data/file/748126/Physical_activity_for_general_health_benefits_in_disabled_adults.pdf

Reid, H., Ridout, J.A., Tomas, S.A., Kelly, P. and Jones, K. (2022). *Benefits outweigh the risks: a consensus statement on the risks of physical activity for people living with long-term conditions*. Available at: https://bjsm.bmj.com/content/early/2021/12/01/bjsports-2021-104281

Richmond Charities. (2016). *People with long term conditions and attitudes to physical activity.* Available at: https://richmondgroupofcharities.org.uk/sites/default/files/richmond_group_debrief_final_1.pdf

Sallis, R., Young, D.R., Tartof, S.Y., Sallis, J., Sall, J., Quiaowu, L., Smith, G. and Cohen, D. (2021). Physical inactivity is associated with A higher risk for severe COVID-19 outcomes: A study in 48 440 adult patients. *British Journal of Sports Medicine*, 55, pp. 1099–1105. Available at: https://bjsm.bmj.com/content/bjsports/55/19/1099.full.pdf

Schuch, F.B., Vancampfort, D., Rosenbaum, S., Richards, J., Ward, P., Veronese, N., Solmi, M., Cadore, E. and Stubbs, B. (2016). Exercise for depression in older adults: A meta-analysis of randomized controlled trials adjusting for publication bias. *Revista Brasileira De Psiquiatria*, 38(3), pp. 247–254. Available at: https://pubmed.ncbi.nlm.nih.gov/27611903/

Sports England. (2017). *Sports outcomes evidence review. Summary of the review of the findings.* Available at: https://sportengland-production-files.s3.eu-west-2.amazonaws.com/s3fs-public/sport-outcomes-evidence-review-report-summary.pdf

Sports England. (2021). *Active lives adult survey May20/21.* Available at: https://sportengland-production-files.s3.eu-west-2.amazonaws.com/s3fs-public/2021-10/Active%20Lives%20Adult%20Survey%20May%202020-21%20Report.pdf?VersionId=YcsnWYZSKx4n12TH0cKpY392hBkRdA8N[

Sports England (2022). *Moving healthcare professionals.* Available at: https://www.sportengland.org/campaigns-and-our-work/moving-healthcare-professionals

Tarp, J., Fagerland, M.W., Dalene, K.E., Morten, W., Johannessen, J., Hansen, Barbara, J.J., Whincup, P.H., Keith, M.D., Hooker, S., Howard, V.J., Chernofsky, A., Larson, M.G., Spartano, N.L., Ramachandran, S.V., Dohrn, I.M., Hagströmer, M., Edwardson, C., Yates, T., Shiroma, E.J., Dempsey, P.C., Wijndaele, K., Anderssen, S.A. and Lee, I.M. and Ekelund, U. (2021). Device-measured physical activity, adiposity and mortality: A harmonised meta-analysis of eight prospective cohort studies. *British Journal of Sports Medicine.* https://doi.org/10.1136/bjsports-2021-104827. PMID: 34876405.

Telama, R., Yang, X., Leskinen, E., Kankaanpää, A., Hirvensalo, M., Tammelin, T., Viikari, J.S. and Raitakari, O.T. (2014). Tracking of physical activity from early childhood through youth into adulthood. *Medicine and Science in Sports and Exercise*, 46(5), pp. 955–962. https://doi.org/10.1249/MSS.0000000000000181.

The Marmot Review. (2010). *Fairer society, healthy lives: Strategic review of health inequalities in England post 2010.* London: Institute of Health Equity. Available at: https://www.instituteofhealthequity.org/resources-reports/fair-society-healthy-lives-the-marmot-review/fair-society-healthy-lives-full-report-pdf.pdf

Tudor-Locke, C., Craig, C.L., Yukitoshi, A., Bell, R., Croteau, K., De Bourdeaudhui, I., Ewald, B., Gardner, A., Hatano, Y., Lutes, L., Matsudo, S., Ramirez-Marrero, F., Rogers, R. and Schmidt, L. S. (2011). How many steps/day are enough? For older adults and special populations. *International Journal of Behavioral Nutrition Physical Activity*, 8, p. 80. https://doi.org/10.1186/1479-5868-8-80.

Wen, C.P. and Wu, X. (2012). Stressing harms of physical inactivity to promote exercise. *Lancet*, 380(9838), pp. 192–193. https://doi.org/10.1016/S0140-6736(12)60954-4. PMID: 22818933.

World Health Organization (WHO). (2009). *Global health risks, mortality and burden of disease attributable to selected major risks.* Available at: https://www.who.int/healthinfo/global_burden_disease/GlobalHealthRisks_report_full.pdf

World Health Organization (WHO). (2018). *More active people, healthier world.* Available at: https://www.paho.org/en/documents/global-action-plan-physical-activity-2018-2030-more-active-people-healthier-world

14 Future and Persistent Challenges in Public Health

Susan R. Thompson

Climate Change

Climate change has been described as the most important health determinant we face as a planet. Greenhouse gases from the burning of fossil fuels are predicted to raise the global temperature to at least 1.5 degrees centigrade above pre industrial levels (Ipcc.ch 2022). Climate change will affect all of us to a greater and lesser extent, but those who will be mostly affected are those in developing countries and where subsistence is already marginal. Low-lying areas and small island states such as Bangladesh and the pacific island of Myanmar are at significant risk of inundation due to rising sea levels. In the UK, the average temperature has risen by 0.25 degrees centigrade per decade since the 1960s with summer rainfall decreasing and winter rainfall increasing (Health Protection Agency [HPA] 2012). Droughts, heatwaves and extreme weather events such as flooding are all increasing their frequency year after year. Transport use accounts for 28% of greenhouse gas emissions in the UK, 14% is due to home energy use (Gov.UK 2022) and 10% is from agriculture in the form of methane release from livestock and nitrous oxide from soils (Ahdb.org.uk 2016). In 2019, the UK pledged to become net zero for greenhouse gas emissions by 2050. Much of the UK housing stock in cities was built in the Victorian period and is difficult to bring up to modern standards of insulation and energy efficiency. These houses are generally lived in by the poorer sections of society and so fuel poverty is a real concern. Food insecurity is also a key issue for the world's population as changes in temperature, precipitation and severe weather events destroy crops and increase prices on the global market, resulting in poorer countries being unable to feed themselves (Wfp.org 2022). In 2021, representatives from countries around the world gathered in Glasgow UK for the 26th COP conference on climate change. Commitments were made for wealthier nations to aid the funding of technological climate change initiatives in the developing world, reduce carbon dioxide emissions by 45% by 2030 and to net zero by 2050, instigate measures to protect ecosystems and acknowledge the need for transition plans to ensure economic stability and job protection. It also acknowledged that previous agreements for action had not been met by all nations signing up to them and encouraged countries to honour their pledges (CP 26 2021). Individually, we can all help by reducing our waste and pressure on resources, saving energy, reducing motor and air transport use, eating less meat and dairy and trying to eat more seasonally rather than buying food which has travelled across the world (Imperial.ac.uk 2013). Following the COVID-19 lockdowns, there was much debate as to how this had affected CO_2 levels in the atmosphere. Research has shown that whilst levels reduced by 7% in 2020, 93% of our normal CO_2 emissions continued and the level of CO_2 in the atmosphere continued to rise (Met Office 2021; Rasmussen 2021). However, models are showing that reducing CO_2

DOI: 10.4324/9781003411321-14

emissions by even a small amount over time will have a cooling effect on the atmosphere (Met Office 2021) in the long term. So we need to learn lessons and resist measures to take us back to the way life was lived before, especially regarding transport use.

Air Pollution

Air pollution is associated with negative health outcomes across the lifespan. Those individuals with existing respiratory illnesses and CVD are particularly susceptible to poor air quality but air pollution has widespread effects. Pregnant women are more likely to give birth to babies with a low birth weight, lung development in children is slowed and in adults pollution contributes to and worsens chronic disease and has been associated with dementia onset (Chief Medical Officer 2022). Outdoor sources are mainly diesel exhausts, burning of fossil fuels and industrial processes including waste incineration, whereas indoor sources include use of kerosene and solid fuels for cooking. Young children, older people and those with chronic conditions are especially at risk (Royal College of Physicians [RCP] 2016). The situation is worse in lower and middle income countries, with 97% of large urban districts in these areas failing to meet World Health Organization (WHO) guidelines on air pollution. However, in 2018, six European countries, namely, France, Germany, Hungary, Italy, Romania and the UK, were all charged with failing to tackle illegal levels of air pollution (WHO 2018). In the UK, a third of children grow up in areas with unacceptable levels of air pollution (United Nations International Children's Emergency Fund [UNICEF] 2018). In the USA, a State of the Air report in 2022 stated that 40% of the population was living with unacceptable levels of air pollution (Lung.org 2022). Many countries have made progress in reducing their emissions. Much of the early work on air pollution targeted the biggest sources of emissions. The UK has now shifted its focus to smaller, more domestic sources of pollution, such as small industrial processes and the need to site these away from residential areas, fertiliser use (the main source of ammonia release), cutting coal and wood use in domestic fires as well as banning the sale of diesel and petrol vehicles (Gov.UK 2019). Between 1980 and 2021, the USA reduced the emissions of the six major pollutants by 75% and reduced carbon dioxide levels to the same as they were in 1980, despite significant population and economic growth. However, this still left 102 million people living with pollutants above acceptable levels (US Environmental Protection Agency 2022). Action to reduce air pollution requires efforts from individuals, organisations and governments. Global agreements are needed to promote cleaner transport and energy generation, better waste management and industrial processes and a reduction in the use of fossil fuels. Better consideration of the urban environment is required to reduce car use and the adoption of green planting schemes which can absorb particulate matter. As children are particularly at risk from air pollution, thought needs to be given to limiting car use near schools, schools could be sited away from busy roads and green space barriers incorporated in planning schemes. Individually, we can use our cars less, reduce our speed and ideally switch to electric vehicles; stop burning coal and wood and insulate our homes to improve energy efficiency.

Food Security

Food security is a growing area of concern worldwide. Food security was defined by the World Food Summit in 1996 as existing when

> all people, at all times, have physical and economic access to sufficient, safe and nutritious food that meets their dietary needs and food preferences for an active and healthy life.
> (World Food Summit 1996)

Climate change crises, domestic food price inflation and the war in Ukraine severely affecting grain exports and increasing energy prices resulted in the world's food import bill rising by 10% in 2022 compared with 2021 prices. This situation has led the Food and Agriculture Organisation of the United Nation to identify 'hunger hotspots', countries where rising prices will drive millions into poverty, hunger and malnourishment. Unsurprisingly the majority of these hotspots are in Africa, but Yemen, Syria, Pakistan and Afghanistan, areas of conflict and insecurity, have also been identified (Food and Agriculture Organization of the United Nations [FAO]-WFP 2022). Economic measures undertaken by governments to control inflation have also compounded the situation, with credit becoming more expensive and food aid decreasing at the time it should be prioritised. Funding for long-term solutions as well as short-term direct food aid is being provided by agencies such as The World Bank, The World Food Programme and others with the aim of facilitating trade to boost supply as well as domestic production and crucially investing in climate-resilient agriculture (The World Bank 2022). Unfortunately, food security is not just a problem for developing nations; deprived communities in developed nations are also finding it hard. The UK in recent years has seen a growth in community organised food banks for those in need. Besides inflation, the blame has been put on the prevalence of low paid work, which means although adults in the family are working, basic necessities are still a struggle. Children without access to regular good nutrition will suffer from poor health and development and lack of educational attainment (Watson and Lloyd 2022). It seems a disgrace that wealthy nations should have to rely on charitable institutions to feed their people. Food banks are in essence subsidising a low wage economy. There are also issues with the food that is provided by these organisations. Pragmatically these small community food banks are housed in local community settings, not refrigerated tailor-made premises such as large supermarkets. This means that the food stored there is largely limited to non-perishable items, canned and packaged food dominate. Research into the nutritional nature of these foodstuffs has shown that they generally have a very high carbohydrate content, especially sugars, and have been seen to be low in certain vitamins, especially vitamins A and D (Fallaize et al. 2020; Oldroyd et al. 2022). Such over reliance on such sources of food will only compound the existing obesity crisis amongst these deprived groups. They are certainly not a long-term solution to food insecurity.

Zoonosis (Infectious Diseases Passing from Animals to Humans)

The 2020–2022 COVID-19 pandemic brought infectious disease back to the forefront of public health departments that, especially in developed countries, had moved away from a need to concentrate on short-term infectious disease onto more chronic long-term disease processes. There has been much debate around the origin of the SARS-CoV-2 virus (COVID-19). The first cases were detected late in 2019 in the Huanan Seafood Market in Wuhan, China. Various speculations took hold, from laboratory leaks to bats, but subsequent research is suggesting that the most likely explanation is that the virus leapt to humans from one or more wild animals which are regularly sold at the market (Science.org 2022). This mechanism is termed zoonosis which the WHO defines as 'any infection which is naturally transmissible from vertebrate animals to humans' (WHO 2020). These pathogens can be parasitic, viral or bacterial and can spread via direct contact, through food, water or contact with the environment of the animals infected. Zoonosis is surprisingly common with some estimates that six out of ten infectious diseases are capable of spreading from animal to humans and perhaps more worrying that three out of four new emerging infectious diseases in humans come from animals (Centers for Disease Control [CDC] 2022; WHO 2020). Examples of such diseases include Ebola, Avian and Swine Flu, Salmonella, HIV and Monkeypox, but it is estimated that there are 200 examples of zoonosis (WHO 2020). The widespread use of antibiotics in farming compounds the problem leading to anti-microbial resistance which is when germs exposed to frequent antibiotics and other drugs are able to adapt themselves to become resistant to their use, making the drugs no longer effective in fighting disease. This is a growing problem worldwide, causing millions of deaths every year and increasing the urgency to discover new more effective drugs (European Medicines Agency [EMA] 2018). Measures to combat zoonosis include ensuring good sanitation and water supply, adherence to food preparation guidelines, effective hand washing especially after contact with animals or their environment, measures to prevent infection from vectors of disease such as ticks and mosquitos and quick reporting and investigation of causes of outbreaks of disease (CDC 2022). It has become evident that despite this being the area of origin, those countries in East and South East Asia that instigated quarantines and lockdowns at the start of the COVID-19 pandemic managed to contain the spread of the virus more effectively than North America, parts of Europe and the UK that delayed lockdowns. The presence of a robust track and trace testing service was also essential in limiting deaths. To this end, the UK, despite being one of the first countries to develop a test for the disease, fell down. The decision to stop its track and trace system early on in the outbreak and instead accept that herd immunity would limit the disease has been shown to have been a grave mistake (Parliament.uk 2021). COVID-19 has illustrated that emerging disease needs to be identified, international cooperation quickly established and measures put in place as early as possible to limit future catastrophes.

Anti-microbial Resistance

As stated above, anti-microbial resistance is a serious and growing health concern. It is estimated that microbes resistant to known drugs are contributing annually to up to 5 million deaths worldwide (Murray et al. 2022). Antibiotics were the wonder drug of the twentieth century. Prior to their discovery, any little infected cut or graze, any episode of tonsillitis or any routine surgical operation had the potential to kill due to the susceptibility of the body to bacterial infection. Later in the century, antivirals were developed which further added to the fight against dangerous microbes. Unfortunately, microbes are clever and by being exposed to anti-microbial drugs over a significant period of time, they have the ability to adapt and dodge the bullets aimed at them. Overuse in humans, animals and plants is largely to blame, unnecessary prescriptions for drugs to treat minor infections that the immune system is capable of combatting on its own. But more action is needed to combat causes of infectious diseases. More preventative work, for example, the provision of clean and safe drinking water, adherence to good food hygiene practices, better sanitation, animal husbandry and agricultural management, would stop infections starting in the first place and remove the need for anti-microbial drugs (WHO 2021). Meanwhile, drug companies are frantically searching for new anti-microbial drugs or different ways of combatting infections. Recent research into peptides, naturally occurring proteins in the body, is looking promising (National Institutes of Health [NIH] 2021).

Gambling

In 2005, the then Labour government in the UK relaxed the laws on gambling (UK Government 2005), making it more accessible than ever before in UK society, whether online, on television or face to face. In 2012, the Commons Culture, Media and Sport Committee published a report looking into changes that had occurred as a result of the act. It concluded that 'Gambling is now widely accepted in the UK as a legitimate entertainment activity' and that the committee opted to 'support liberalisation of rules' (Commons Select Committee 2012). In 2021, a report into the level of gambling in UK society showed that 30.5 million adults or 59% of the population had gambled in some form within the last 12-month period, with 13% or 6.5 million of these being classed as problem gamblers (YouGov 2021). Sustained gambling over a period of hours has been seen to greatly increase stress levels resulting in increased heart rate and cortisol levels and has been thought to cause cardiac arrest (Meyer et al. 2000). These are the short-term health effects. Sustained problem gambling can cause family breakdown, domestic violence, criminal activity, loss and disruption to employment and social isolation. Money spent on gambling means less money for everyday essentials of life such as good housing, nutrition and payment of utility bills. It is estimated that for every individual who has a problem with gambling, five to ten others in contact with that individual suffer the repercussions of the gambler's habit (Public Health England [PHE] 2021). Problem gamblers have typically been shown to have a higher alcohol consumption, worse mental health and are 19 times more likely to die from suicide than those who do not gamble (PHE 2021).

All forms of gambling have seen an increase in recent years and problem gamblers are more likely to be middle-aged males, although women are also affected especially through their use of online slot machines. Those living in deprived areas were also disproportionately affected, with 20% of the poorest regions in the UK providing 25% of the industry's £10 billion profits (National Centre for Social Research 2022). Advertising of gambling has increased dramatically in recent years, with the industry currently spending £1.5 billion a year in the UK (House of Lords Library 2022). This situation has seen increasing calls for tighter controls on the gambling industry. Although gambling organisations have a duty to identify and support problem gamblers, in 2022 a major player was fined £17 million by the UK government for failing to protect its vulnerable customers, although this amounted to just 3% of that company's previous year's revenue.

In 2020, the UK government launched a review of the 2005 Gambling Act. Its aim was to update regulations in light of the digital age, examine support provided for problem gamblers, consider gambling advertising and ways to cut down on illegal operations (UK Parliament 2022). The publication of this review has been delayed four times, with the speculation that this is due to pressure from the gambling industry which is resistant to further regulation (All Party Parliamentary Betting and Gaming Group [APBGG] 2022). However, all party groups and the House of Lords have called for greater regulation in the form of greater powers for the Gambling Commission to: withdraw licences from operators, regularly conduct affordability checks on customers, a levy on the industry to fund research into gambling, more restriction on advertising especially sports sponsorship and an independent ombudsman to resolve disputes between customers and gambling organisations (House of Lords Library 2022). It remains to be seen whether the review supports these proposals.

References

Ahdb.org.uk. (2016). *Carbon: greenhouse gas emissions from agriculture | AHDB* [online]. Available at: https://ahdb.org.uk/carbon

All Party Parliamentary Betting and Gaming Group (APBGG). (2022). *All Party Parliamentary Betting and Gaming Group*. https://www.apbgg.org/

Centers for Disease Control (CDC). (2022). *Zoonotic diseases*. [online] Available at: https://www.cdc.gov/onehealth/basics/zoonotic-diseases.html

Chief Medical Officer. (2022). *Annual report: Air pollution.* Available at: https://www.gov.uk/government/publications/chief-medical-officers-annual-report-2022-air-pollution

Commons Select Committee. (2012). *The Gambling Act 2005, a bet worth taking?*

CP 26. (2021). *Glasgow Climate Pact. Decision* [online] Available at: https://unfccc.int/sites/default/files/resource/cop26_auv_2f_cover_decision.pdf

European Medicines Agency (EMA). (2018). *Antimicrobial resistance - European Medicines Agency* [online]. European Medicines Agency. Available at: https://www.ema.europa.eu/en/human-regulatory/overview/public-health-threats/antimicrobial-resistance

Fallaize, R., Newlove, J., White, A. and Lovegrove, J.A. (2020). Nutritional adequacy and content of food bank parcels in Oxfordshire, UK: A comparative analysis of independent and organisational provision. *Journal of Human Nutrition and Dietetics* [online], 33(4), pp. 477–486. doi: 10.1111/jhn.12740.

Food and Agriculture Organization of the United Nations (FAO). (2022). Food and Agriculture Organisation of the United Nations and World Food Programme. *Hunger Hotspots, FAO-WFP Early warning on acute food insecurity October 2022 – Jan 2023 outlook.* FAO-WFP. Rome. Available at: https://docs.wfp.org/api/documents/WFP-0000142656/download/?_ga=2.114821124.2083527230.1671206557-287562329.1664360267

Gov.UK. (2019). *Clean air strategy.* Available at: https://assets.publishing.service.gov.uk/government/uploads/system/uploads/attachment_data/file/770715/clean-air-strategy-2019.pdf

Gov.UK. (2022). *UK Climate Change Risk Assessment 2022* [online]. Gov.UK. Available at: https://www.gov.uk/government/publications/uk-climate-change-risk-assessment-2022

Health Protection Agency (HPA). (2012). *Health Effects of Climate Change in the UK 2012 Current evidence, recommendations and research gaps* [online]. Available at: https://assets.publishing.service.gov.uk/government/uploads/system/uploads/attachment_data/file/371103/Health_Effects_of_Climate_Change_in_the_UK_2012_V13_with_cover_accessible.pdf

House of Lords Library. (2022). *How should gambling regulation change to reduce gambling harm?* [online]. House of Lords Library. Available at: https://lordslibrary.parliament.uk/how-should-gambling-regulation-change-to-reduce-gambling-harm/

Imperial.ac.uk. (2022). *9 things you can do about climate change* [online]. Available at: https://www.imperial.ac.uk/stories/climate-action/

Ipcc.ch. (2022). *Climate Change 2022: Impacts, adaptation and vulnerability* [online]. Available at: https://www.ipcc.ch/report/ar6/wg2/

Lung.org. (2022). *Key findings | State of the air* [online]. Available at: https://www.lung.org/research/sota/key-findings

Met Office. (2021). *How did COVID-19 lockdowns affect the climate?* [online]. Available at: https://www.metoffice.gov.uk/research/news/2021/how-did-covid-19-lockdowns-affect-the-climate#:~:text=Gases%20like%20carbon%20dioxide%20have,levels%20continued%20to%20build%20up

Meyer, G., Hauffa, B.P., Schedlowski, M., Pawluk, C., Stadler, M.A. and Exton, M.S. (2000). Casino gambling increases heart rate and salivary cortisol in regular gamblers. *Biological Psychiatry*, 48, pp. 948–953.

Murray, C.J., Ikuta, K.S., Sharara, F., Swetschinski, L., Robles Aguilar, G., Gray, A., Han, C., Bisignano, C., Rao, P., Wool, E., Johnson, S.C., Browne, A.J., Chipeta, M.G., Fell, F., Hackett, S., Haines-Woodhouse, G., Kashef Hamadani, B.H., Kumaran, E.A.P., McManigal, B. and Agarwal, R. (2022). Global burden of bacterial antimicrobial resistance in 2019: A systematic analysis. *The Lancet* [online], 399(10325), pp. 629–655. doi: 10.1016/s0140-6736(21)02724-0.

National Centre for Social Research. (2022). *Patterns of play.* NatCen Social Research.

National Institutes of Health (NIH). (2021). *Searching for new antibiotics in the human body* [online]. Available at: https://www.nih.gov/news-events/nih-research-matters/searching-new-antibiotics-human-body

Oldroyd, L., Eskandari, F., Pratt, C. and Lake, A.A. (2022). The nutritional quality of food parcels provided by food banks and the effectiveness of food banks at reducing food insecurity in developed countries: A mixed-method systematic review. *Journal of Human Nutrition and Dietetics* [online], 35(6), pp. 1202–1229. doi: 10.1111/jhn.12994.

Parliament.uk. (2021). *Coronavirus: lessons learned to date report published - Committees - UK Parliament* [online]. Available at: https://committees.parliament.uk/committee/81/health-and-social-care-committee/news/157991/coronavirus-lessons-learned-to-date-report-published/

Public Health England (PHE). (2021). *Risk factors for gambling and harmful gambling: An umbrella review* [online]. Available at: https://assets.publishing.service.gov.uk/government/uploads/system/uploads/attachment_data/file/1020749/Gambling_risk_factors.pdf

Rasmussen, C. (2021). *Emission reductions from pandemic had unexpected effects on atmosphere* [online]. Climate Change: Vital Signs of the Planet. Available at: https://climate.nasa.gov/news/3129/emission-reductions-from-pandemic-had-unexpected-effects-on-atmosphere/

Royal College of Physicians (RCP). (2016). *Every breathe we take, the lifelong impact of air pollution.* London: Royal College of Physicians.

Science.org. (2022). *Evidence suggests pandemic came from nature not a lab panel says.* Available at: https://www.science.org/content/article/evidence-suggests-pandemic-came-nature-not-lab-panel-says

The World Bank. (2022). *Food security update.* Available at: https://www.worldbank.org/en/topic/agriculture/brief/food-security-update

UK Government. (2005). *Gambling Act 2005* [online]. Available at: https://www.legislation.gov.uk/ukpga/2005/19/contents

UK Parliament. (2022). *Gambling-related harm* [online]. House of Commons Library. Available at: https://commonslibrary.parliament.uk/research-briefings/cdp-2022-0071/#:~:text=The%20Government's%20Review%20of%20the,are%20considering%20the%20evidence%20carefully.

United Nations International Children's Emergency Fund (UNICEF). (2018). *A breath of toxic air.* https://www.unicef.org.uk/publications/child-health-breah-of-toxic-air/

US Environmental Protection Agency. (2022). *Air quality - National summary | US EPA* [online]. Available at: https://www.epa.gov/air-trends/air-quality-national-summary#:~:text=In%202021%2C%20about%2067%20million,of%20acids%2C%20and%20visibility%20impairment.

Watson, M.C. and Lloyd, J. (2022). Food banks should be phased out: Fiscal measures are needed. *British Medical Journal Rapid Response*, 11th December 2022. https://www.bmj.com/content/379/bmj.o2919/rr

Wfp.org. (2022). *A global food crisis | World Food Programme* [online]. Available at: https://www.wfp.org/global-hunger-crisis.

World Food Summit. (1996). *Final Report.* Available at: https://www.fao.org/3/w3548e/w3548e00.htm

World Health Organization (WHO). (2018). *Household air pollution and health.* Geneva: WHO. https://www.who.int/news-room/fact-sheets/detail/household-air-pollution-and-health

World Health Organization (WHO). (2020). *Health topics: Zoonosis.* Geneva. Available at: https://www.who.int/news-room/fact-sheets/detail/zoonoses#:~:text=A%20zoonosis%20is%20an%20infectious,food%2C%20water%20or%20the%20environment

World Health Organization (WHO). (2021). *WHO strategic priorities on antimicrobial resistance: Preserving antimicrobials for today and tomorrow.* Available at: WHO Strategic Priorities on Antimicrobial Resistance

YouGov. (2021). *Annual GB treatment and support survey 2021 of behalf of GambleAware.* Available at: https://www.begambleaware.org/sites/default/files/2022-03/Annual%20GB%20Treatment%20and%20Support%20Survey%20Report%202021%20%28FINAL%29_0.p

Glossary

Asylum Seeker A person who has left their country of origin and lodged an application for asylum in another country and is waiting for the results of that application.

Comparative Needs Needs which arise from the requirement to ensure equity of provision to similar populations.

Epidemiology The study of disease and health determinants within populations.

Expressed Needs Needs identified from the level of use of services already provided.

Felt Needs The health needs that are identified by people themselves.

Health Impact Assessment Investigations into the possible negative wider ramifications of proposed interventions.

Health Literacy The level of knowledge of health issues and their determinants possessed by communities or individuals and their capacity to act on these.

Incidence The number of **new** cases of a certain condition appearing in a population.

Index of Multiple Deprivation (IMD) A measurement used to score the level of deprivation of local authority areas in the UK.

Intersectionality Multiple intersecting factors of advantage or disadvantage affecting the health of individuals.

Inverse Care 'Law' The acknowledged fact that the more needy and deprived a person is the less care they receive and vice versa.

Models Frameworks based on best practice which act as tools for health promoters to use to ensure effective working.

Morbidity Suffering from a state of ill health, either physical or mental, as a result of a disease, illness or injury.

Motivational Interviewing A person centred method of supporting individuals through behaviour change.

Normative Needs Health needs of a population decided upon by professionals as a result of studying epidemiological trends.

Peer Education Utilisation of community members who have commonality with the target population, e.g. breastfeeding counsellors and community nutrition assistants.

Prevalence The number of cases of a certain condition present in a population at a certain time.

Proportionate Universalism Although preventative health services will be available to all, to combat health inequalities those who are disadvantaged in society will receive a greater proportion of these services.

Protected Characteristics Nine characteristics identified by the UK Equality and Human Rights Commission which are liable to be the focus of discrimination and should therefore be protected. These are discrimination on the grounds of age, gender, disability,

666666666666

sexual orientation, gender reassignment, civil partnerships, race, pregnancy and maternity, religion and belief.

Refugee   According to The 1951 UN Convention on Refugees, someone 'owing to a well-founded fear of being persecuted for reasons of race, religion, nationality, membership of a particular social group, or political opinion, is outside the country of his nationality, and is unable to or, owing to such fear, is unwilling to avail himself of the protection of that country or who, not having a nationality and being outside the country of his former habitual residence as a result of such events, is unable or, owing to such fear, is unwilling to return to it'. Those granted refugee status have a right to remain in the country granting it.

Self-Efficacy   An individual's belief that they will have the motivation and ability to undertake successful behaviour change.

Sensitivity (of screening test)   The level of which the test is able to detect **all** those which the disease or trait that test is designed to detect.

Specificity (of screening test)   The level of which the test accurately detects **only those** with the disease or trait being screened for.

Social Capital   The level of involvement by individuals in the life of their community and their commitment to it.

Social Epidemiology   The study of the social factors which influence health.

Social Gradient of Health   The term describing that the lower a person's level is in society, the worse their health.

Social Marketing   The use of advertising industry techniques to persuade individuals to change their attitudes and behaviour.

Social Prescribing   Referral often by health professionals to activities seen as a means of improving the individual's physical or mental health status. Examples are green gyms, garden schemes, exercise on prescription and community projects.

Stakeholders   Agencies, organisations and client groups with a connection to a particular health issue or community.

Standardised Mortality Ratio (SMR)   The SMR is used to compare the mortality risk of a study population to that of a standard population. The standard population is stated as 100. Therefore, a figure of under 100 for a specific population suggests less than expected deaths, whereas a figure of over 100 indicates more than expected deaths. SMR is often used to compare different geographical areas and population groups.

Index